Adrenal

Fatigue

Step-by-step Guide How to Overcome
Adrenal Fatigue

*(Save Your Life & Career with Holistic Secrets to
Naturally Reclaim Your Energy)*

Antonio Castro

Published By **Chris David**

Antonio Castro

All Rights Reserved

Adrenal Fatigue: Step-by-step Guide How to Overcome Adrenal Fatigue (Save Your Life & Career with Holistic Secrets to Naturally Reclaim Your Energy)

ISBN 978-1-998927-85-2

Legal & Disclaimer

The information contained in this book is not designed to replace or take the place of any form of medicine or professional medical advice. The information in this book has been provided for educational & entertainment purposes only.

The information contained in this book has been compiled from sources deemed reliable, and it is accurate to the best of the Author's knowledge; however, the Author cannot guarantee its accuracy and validity and cannot be held liable for any errors or omissions. Changes are periodically made to this book. You must consult your doctor or get professional medical advice before using any of the suggested remedies, techniques, or information in this book.

Table Of Contents

Chapter 1: About Adrenal Glands & Hormone Production

Before we get to the good things to help you heal Adrenal Fatigue manifestly, it's essential to first recognize what the adrenal glands are, how they paintings, and what characteristic they play in a healthy-functioning body. It's a touch in depth, but undergo with me. This will assist you higher understand why and the way some of the treatments I propose art work.

Adrenal glands are a key detail of what's referred to as the HPA Axis: the hypothalamus, pituitary, and the adrenal glands. These three glands artwork together in a feedback loop to control and modify metabolism and power tiers, libido, immune gadget, mood and stress reaction.

Hypothalamus

The hypothalamus, located deep within the forebrain, produces and secretes the hormone "corticotrophin-liberating issue", or CRF, in reaction to pressure. The extra stress, the more CRF is generated by way of the hypothalamus.

Pituitary

The pituitary sits beneath the hypothalamus. As the hypothalamus secretes CRF, it stimulates the pituitary to release adrenocorticotropic hormone (ACTH), which travels to the adrenals and kidneys.

Adrenals

The adrenals are walnut-sized glands placed just above each of the kidneys and they play a massive position to your popular fitness. (The root of the phrase "adrenal" comes from the Latin "advert", or near, and "renes", it really is kidney.) They respond to the messages from the pituitary by means of way of producing hormones or chemical materials that modify the metabolism, infection and immune response.

Each adrenal gland is created from terrific additives, with super abilities.

Adrenal Cortex

This is the outer layer, or shell, of the gland. Its undertaking is to offer hormones which have an impact on metabolism and special chemical materials within the blood.

Cortisol

Cortisol is one of the stars of the glucocorticoid family. Cortisol is famous for triggering our physical pressure response to melancholy, anxiety, and further exercise, loss of sleep or trauma. Cortisol stimulates norepinephrine, sometimes known as noradrenaline, to vicinity the frame into "fight or flight" mode. I will deal with extra about cortisol in a 2d.

Aldosterone

Aldosterone regulates potassium and sodium levels, and facilitates to keep blood stress and blood quantity.

Androgenic Steroids (Androgen Hormones)

The androgenic hormones, such as DHEA (dehydroepiandrosterone), produced in the adrenal cortex are transformed into female hormones (estrogen) or male hormones (androgens and testosterone), and they will be additionally produced a few vicinity else in the body in massive quantities.

Adrenal Medulla

This inner middle of the adrenal gland is chargeable for generating the hormones that help us address emotional and bodily strain.

Epinephrine (Adrenaline)

Epinephrine lets in blood float to the muscle tissues and the mind, permits convert glycogen to glucose inside the liver, and will boom each the coronary heart rate and the pressure of coronary heart contractions.

Norepinephrine (Noradrenaline)

This is the hormone that outcomes in vasoconstriction, the squeezing of the blood vessels, which allows hold or increase blood stress even as in acute stress.

Cortisol Hormone

Cortisol, the stress hormone, is the most crucial hormone inside the body's response to stress. Cortisol permits maintain the frame in stability, called homeostasis, with the aid of moderating or regulating activation of the precious concerned tool, anti-inflammatory and immune responses, glucose or blood sugar degrees, blood vessel and coronary coronary heart contractions and tone, and as referenced in advance, the metabolism of fat, protein and carbohydrates.

If it's miles crucial for the adrenals to offer extra cortisol in response to pressure, it's far similarly essential for frame competencies and cortisol stages to variety and move back to a normal u . S . A . After the annoying event has passed. This is in element what gets lessen to rubble with Adrenal Fatigue Syndrome.

In our excessive-strain tradition, regularly the times of our lives don't generate this "pass again to regular" sign up that HPA axis comments loop.

When the adrenals end up overworked, producing an excessive amount of cortisol, they begin to show off signs and signs and symptoms and signs and symptoms of harm and tear, not capable of hold up with the call for. When this takes place, cortisol ranges drop and the frame and mind are no longer capable of efficiently respond to traumatic or excessive-strain situations.

Connection to the Thyroid

The thyroid and cortisol hormones have a totally close to dating. They art work in tandem to ensure the body has sufficient power. Hypothyroidism, wherein the thyroid doesn't produce sufficient thyroid hormone, is a very not unusual state of affairs. Prescription capsules can also assist repair the thyroid stability in plenty of sufferers, but not in all. In sufferers who do not reply to this supply of bio-identical or desiccated thyroid, the symptoms of thoughts fog, tension, strain and coffee energy regularly persist. The lacking link is regularly Adrenal Fatigue.

Chapter 2: What Is Adrenal Fatigue?

Based on what you've take a look at thus far, you'll understand that it's a pressure scenario. Adrenal Fatigue is an umbrella term for a set of signs and signs and signs which might be because of the adrenal glands now not strolling at their most beneficial, and as a cease cease end result, they fail to offer sufficient portions of vital hormones wished via manner of the body. When the adrenals prevent acting nicely, all elements of the frame are affected.

In healthy, low-stress humans, the remarks loop of the HPA axis works harmoniously. But, at the same time as there is chronic overproduction of cortisol and norepinephrine, the machine turns into desensitized, or immune, to the terrible messages to "sit back out". This is what eventually consequences in continual stress on all three glands and often results in a number of fatigue situations.

The overwhelming fundamental symptom of Adrenal Fatigue is fatigue, mainly with problem waking up within the morning. You might also moreover revel in weight benefit or issue losing weight, sudden or abrupt weight reduction, cravings for candy or salty substances, hair loss, low blood strain, recurrent infections and sluggish recuperation.

We'll get into extra detail approximately the signs and symptoms and signs and symptoms and signs and symptoms and symptoms of Adrenal Fatigue in Chapter four.

What Causes Adrenal Fatigue?

Western society is more and more speedy-paced, and it's far actually more difficult than it modified into, even 50 years inside the past, to take a destroy and rest. Not just bodily, but emotionally and mentally. Things like generation, in which our gadgets follow a whole lot people to mattress, career pressures, dating and circle of relatives troubles, can all upload as plenty as generate a steady circulate of pressure. At a fine point lots of us forestall being capable of correctly reply whilst heightened or extreme strain occasions occur, and occasionally this results in an loss of functionality to cope or function with the stresses of ordinary dwelling.

Boiled proper down to basics, stress causes Adrenal Fatigue. Your adrenal glands truly become a whole lot much less and much much less able to cope with the hormone-manufacturing needs strain is placing on them.

What motives Adrenal Fatigue in one man or woman may be quite super from the motive in every other. Pinpointing the exact motive can be difficult. The signs and signs and symptoms and signs and symptoms and symptoms make bigger slowly, on occasion over a decade or more. It isn't uncommon for a person to undergo Adrenal Fatigue

Syndrome and never truly realize precisely what the cause changed into. There are some of reasons that may be grouped into six number one lessons, in no particular order:

#1: Trauma

A single, physically stressful occasion can reason Adrenal Fatigue, which sometimes manifests years later. Car accidents, most essential surgical treatment, severe sports activities activities activities injuries or distinct events all fall into this elegance.

#2: Chronic Disease

Coping with continual contamination or disease locations above-everyday goals to your adrenal glands. Fibromyalgia, chronic ache, Lyme illness, bronchial hypersensitive reactions, diabetes or arthritis may additionally all be factors.

#three: Not Enough Sleep

Most contemporary surveys advocate Americans have become an average of simply over 6 hours of sleep in line with night time time. That's down from an average of eight hours of sleep every night time 50 to one hundred years inside the beyond, and quick of the 8 – nine hours of relaxation the professionals recommend we want earlier than we are prone to growing sleep issues and unique related illnesses.

#four: Emotional Stress

Different from the pressure due to physical trauma, emotional strain can also moreover additionally sense viable in the brief term. However, prolonged periods under emotional stress can reason, or at the least make a contribution to, Adrenal Fatigue. Whether it's a awful boss at paintings, an sad courting, having a sick little one, transferring, or the demise of a family member, emotional stress can turn out to be persistent if the underlying cause isn't dealt with.

#five: Poor Diet, Crash Dieting & Addictions

You've heard the pronouncing 'you're what you eat'. Unhealthy ingesting styles that include too much fast food, immoderate delicate sugar and fat consumption, and yo-yo or crash weight loss program all located a notable stress at the adrenal glands as they warfare to hold homeostasis within the body. Addictions to alcohol, pills, and eating problems will all purpose your adrenals to art work more difficult and could boom the threat they will turn out to be fatigued.

#6: Pollutants and Chemicals (Addictions)

'Toxic load' is a word used to explain the overall degree of toxicity in our environments. Air pollutants (from motors, organization), antibiotics in meat, insecticides on end result and greens, even chlorine in our eating water. All of those, and extra, are chemical compounds that might have a cloth and terrible effect on our everyday fitness, together with the adrenals. Some of these chemical materials without a doubt disrupt adrenal feature, forcing the opposite factors of the HPA axis to alter and fill the void.

Four Levels of Adrenal Fatigue

All Adrenal Fatigue isn't always the equal and symptoms can range extensively among humans. In a unmarried individual the type and diploma of signs and symptoms and signs and symptoms and signs can trade through the years. What I've positioned, even though, is that there are commonly 4 distinctive ranges of Adrenal Fatigue, and those stages represent the development method of adrenal exhaustion.

Level One: Initial Stress Response

This is the number one section of pressure response, at some point of which the body stays making enough of the hormones needed to correctly respond to a pressure cause. Blood tests administered on the equal time as in this diploma would possibly display better degrees of cortisol, adrenaline, norepinephrine, insulin and DHEA.

It's ordinary for us to slip outside and inside of degree one severa instances in the course of our lives, and at the same time as sleep also can additionally begin to go through, signs and symptoms and symptoms are rarely bothersome enough to file or looking for treatment.

Level Two: Alarm

Alarm bells start to ring as the endocrine gadget starts offevolved offevolved to divert belongings from sex hormone manufacturing over to strain hormone manufacturing. In diploma there is often a persistent feeling of being worn-out however hyper-alert: daylight alertness to characteristic usually with a fatigue crash inside the midnight. Unhealthy dependence on caffeine or alcohol and specific materials regularly develops inside the alarm diploma.

Level Three: Resistance

The frame demonstrates its brilliance in degree , adapting to extended pressure through generating extra strain hormones and less sex hormones. Testosterone and DHEA degrees drop in order that the endocrine device can hold generating more cortisol. Life and project characteristic frequently however seem regular on the identical time as in degree three, but fundamental symptoms along with decreased sex energy, ordinary infections and tiredness start to take their toll.

A character can hang around in 'resistance' territory for months, and every so often even years.

Level Four: Burnout

All the assets used to divert hormone manufacturing to cortisol production are used up, or maybe cortisol levels start to drop. Low intercourse hormones, low pressure hormones, and occasional neurotransmitters too. It's the crash that regularly arrives after lengthy intervals of big pressure. Here the symptoms may be stated finally of the frame: excessive fatigue, apathy, depression, tension, weight loss, and despair, to name only some. In burnout, you may frequently discover that you can't hold up with the normal pace that has been "everyday" in your life to this point. Recovery from burnout regularly calls for a whole life-style alternate, alongside aspect healthy doses of each persistence and time.

Chapter 3: Overlooked, Misdiagnosed, Misunderstood

Adrenal Fatigue is quite arguable. The medical network is break up as to whether or not or now not there is a scientific basis for a diagnosis of Adrenal Fatigue, and lots of argue there may be top notch scientifically demonstrated diagnoses to provide an purpose for Adrenal Fatigue signs and symptoms and signs and symptoms and signs.

It's actual there are a number of one-of-a-kind illnesses that can be related to Adrenal Fatigue: fibromyalgia, continual fatigue syndrome, hypothyroidism, estrogen dominance, ovarian-adrenal-thyroid imbalance syndrome, and others. Generalized signs can often overlap. Proponents of Adrenal Fatigue be given as genuine with that during a few times AFS is the underlying purpose of those other conditions. Allow me to attempt to paint a easy image of why I consider this scientific struggle exists.

Adrenal Insufficiency Versus Adrenal Fatigue

Adrenal insufficiency, referred to as Addison's Disease, stocks a number of the signs and symptoms of Adrenal Fatigue, however they will be a good deal extra extreme. Addison's is regularly moreover followed via the use of prolonged vomiting, excessive muscle weakness, very low blood pressure or maybe wonder, profound sleepiness or maybe coma. If you positioned this sounds essential, you're actually correct. A man or woman with those symptoms may be in adrenal disaster and needs emergency medical treatment.

Adrenal insufficiency takes vicinity at the same time as the adrenal glands aren't able to function, inside the event that they're absent or had been eliminated. Most often adrenal insufficiency is the stop result of an autoimmune ailment, in which the body's very very own immune machine assaults the cells of the adrenal glands. Infection, which includes tuberculosis, also can be a purpose. And in times in which the adrenal glands have been surgically removed there is apparent number one adrenal insufficiency.

Taking synthetic steroid medicinal pills like prednisolone, prednisone and dexamethasone also can bring about adrenal insufficiency as it tips the pituitary gland into questioning there can be more than sufficient cortisol inside the bloodstream, so it doesn't inform the adrenals to fabricate any extra.

Endocrinologists warn that via manner of taking adrenal nutritional dietary supplements containing extracts of energetic adrenal hormone unnecessarily can also render the adrenal glands useless and they'll no longer paintings after they're wanted maximum. Many immoderate illnesses, like rheumatic sicknesses, most cancers, hepatitis C and more, percentage symptoms along with fatigue, and self-medicating with those adrenal dietary dietary supplements can also additionally allow the underlying disorder to improvement undetected for too prolonged earlier than detection.

History of Adrenal Fatigue

Once Dr. Thomas Addison first furnished his idea on a sickness of the "suprarenal pills" (in recent times called adrenal glands) that furnished as an anemia-like condition inside the mid-1800s. Subsequently it have become referred to as Addison's Disease. Addison's findings added on in addition studies and caused what have turn out to be the area of endocrinology.

Later that century, physicians began the use of extracts from porcine adrenal cells (yup, pigs) to cope with every Addison's Disease and the milder situation known as hypoadrenia.

"Adrenal Fatigue" as a term commenced growing within the overdue 1990's. That's whilst Dr. James L. Wilson, a naturopath and chiropractor with three PhD's, started out out the usage of it to explain a set of symptoms and symptoms and signs and symptoms that have been comparable throughout some of tired, immune-compromised sufferers.

The debate among specific factions of the medical community over the existence of Adrenal Fatigue has not changed a splendid deal within the final century. What's on the center of this debate? The question of whether or not the street amongst health and contamination is as stable as black and white, wherein a affected man or woman is both sick or healthful, or whether or not there can be whole spectrum on which there are various tiers amongst extensively unwell and honestly healthy.

Illness-Wellness Continuum

In 1972, John W. Travis first proposed the concept of the "contamination-well-being" continuum. Travis, founding father of The Wellness Resource Centre in Mill Valley, California, opined that it want to take appreciably greater than the easy absence of detectable 'contamination' to determine whether or not someone modified into "properly".

On the some distance left of Travis' continuum is early or pre-mature lack of life. In the center is a impartial factor in which there can be no evidence of every contamination or wellness. On the far proper of the continuum is a excessive degree of fitness. And in between the 2 points, from left to right, are:

•Disability

•Symptoms

•Signs

- Neutral (no detectible contamination or wellness)

- Awareness

- Education

- Growth

This continuum, which thru the manner echoes the view of the World Health Organization, contradicts the techniques of health experts that only interact, diagnose and cope with humans at the same time as they'll be in reality unwell, at the left-hand detail of the continuum: that is, displaying signs and symptoms, symptoms and signs and symptoms or even incapacity related to sickness.

Travis moreover believes that the "mind-set" of everyone plays a sizable position in wherein they fall on the continuum. Those with a excellent outlook on life ought to have better fitness effects than those with a terrible outlook on life, no matter the presence or absence of laboratory-confirmed ailment.

Subclinical Versus Clinical

There are many ailments that live beneath the edge of clinical laboratory detection: examples embody rheumatoid arthritis, mild hypothyroidism and diabetes. Adrenal Fatigue is the subclinical syndrome of Adrenal Insufficiency, or Addison's sickness. By the time the laboratory checks "display" adrenal insufficiency, regularly the excellent remedy choice is lifelong alternative of bio-equal corticosteroids.

Diagnostic strategies and laboratory assessments are tremendously mechanized and do not bear in mind the splendid uniqueness of everybody's frame. No real data, no take a look at nutrients, lifestyle or genetic factors thru which to view lab take a look at effects.

Reliance on laboratory take a look at consequences which can be skewed to an all or not anything technique depart no room to keep in mind Adrenal Fatigue Syndrome as subclinical to Addison's Disease, or that mild variations of outcomes within a "ordinary" variety can also simply be signs of horrific adrenal fitness in a few sufferers. Doctors wearing those all or not something blinders condemn sufferers which includes you and me to each go through needlessly or are searching for on our very personal for answers.

Advances in preventive and so-called alternative treatment are helping those sufferers. In typically they're capable of save you ailment improvement at the same time as it's far nonetheless on this "sub-scientific" u . S . A . In order that it does no longer emerge as greater severe.

Large Patient Pool

There is a developing swell of humans which consist of you who're inclined and organized to take their fitness into their very very own arms and look for techniques to help themselves to heal and revel in better. According to Dr. Michael Lam (a Medical Doctor with a Masters of Public Health and certification from the American Board of Anti-Aging Medicine who makes a speciality of Adrenal Fatigue and dietary medication), over 50 percent of the individual populace will suffer from Adrenal Fatigue in a few unspecified time inside the future in their lifetime.

At the time of this writing, 1.45 million searching for effects were once more after getting into "Adrenal Fatigue" into Google's are seeking for engine. That's loads of hobby and interest for a syndrome that conventional treatment doesn't outcomes understand.

There is currently no easy laboratory test that may be select out or affirm a evaluation of Adrenal Fatigue. This is, as a minimum in element, what is at the foundation of the speak, or conflict, among medical and health practitioners over Adrenal Fatigue (and outstanding conditions).

In many patients, laboratory blood exams will turn up "ordinary", leaving the affected man or woman to experience like he or she is "loopy", imagining matters, or a hypochondriac. Don't melancholy if that is taking place, or has passed off, to you! Keep analyzing. I can assist.

 Medical Evolution

Let's do not forget that till very currently, the Western treatment network also didn't recognize chronic fatigue syndrome, fibromyalgia, chiropractors, naturopaths or Chinese medication, which has been practiced for masses of years. We best want to appearance lower back a hundred years or so you ought to locate that "hysteria" become a catchall description for a host of "girl" troubles from fainting to anxiety, sleeplessness to irritability and anxiety, with questionable techniques of remedy. Can it's this shape of stretch to expect that medicinal drug will catch up and Adrenal Fatigue becomes a more extensively recognized syndrome?

As more and more dad and mom take our numerous physical court cases to our clinical medical scientific docs, who tell us "your exams are all terrible", and then keep to do our very own research and take our fitness into our private hands, the scientific community may need to have increasingly more motives to adjust their method.

Chapter 4: Adrenal Fatigue. Do You Have It?

As I just referenced in Chapter 3, different medical conditions can produce the identical signs and symptoms as Adrenal Fatigue. It is important to ensure you've got got recognized, and been handled for, a few distinctive conditions or fitness factors that may be contributing in your signs and signs earlier than reaching a evaluation of Adrenal Fatigue.

Adrenal Fatigue Syndrome provides with a combination of signs and symptoms and symptoms that collectively, together with the absence of every other formal medical diagnosis, brings you to the belief that your adrenal glands are beneath-functioning, or fatigued.

Signs and Symptoms of Adrenal Fatigue

There are common signs and symptoms and signs and symptoms and signs, professional through almost all and sundry with Adrenal

Fatigue in numerous ranges or depth. These are:

•Fatigue

•Weight gain tendency, especially at some stage in the waist

•Frequent flu or specific breathing ailments or infections that ultimate longer than ordinary

•Low intercourse electricity

•Dizziness or lightheadedness on the same time as recognition

•Poor reminiscence and muddled thinking

•Low morning energy, in addition to in the past due afternoon

•Need caffeine or one-of-a-kind stimulants to begin the day

•Meals supply quick remedy

•Food cravings for fatty, salty and sugary factors

•Unexplained neck, top or decrease once more ache

•Increased PMS, with intervals which is probably heavy and save you, or almost prevent, on about day 4, starting yet again on day 5 or 6

•Startle without trouble

•Feeling crushed, trouble managing stress and responsibility

•Body temperature troubles: bloodless arms and feet, warmness face, heat flashes

•Unexplained hair loss, and

•Multiple allergic reactions or sensitivities to food

Physical Signs

Fatigue

Fatigue is the most vital symptom of Adrenal Fatigue, and is gift to three diploma in each affected person with AFS. In unique, upon waking in the morning, irrespective of how long or how specific a sleep you've had, feeling gradual and simply now not capable of "awaken" within the morning is a key symptom.

•Puffy, swollen eyes in the morning,

•Battling fatigue at some point of the day, with a big low inside the late afternoon

•Disrupted sleep, and

•Feeling the maximum energetic inside the nighttime

Weight Gain or Changes, Food Cravings

•Abdominal fat accumulation this is unexplained

•Need for coffee or different stimulants to "get going" within the morning

•Cravings for fatty elements, and

•Cravings for salty or sweet additives

Blood Pressure

•Consistent low blood pressure, and

•Dizziness while getting up from mendacity or sitting

Anxiety

•Inability to relax, notwithstanding fatigue, feeling stressed

•Feelings of low arrogance and despair

•Panic attacks, and

•Feeling of adrenalin rushes

Hormones/Libido

•Low thyroid characteristic (hypothyroidism) that doesn't seem to reply to medication, and

•Low sex energy

Female Issues

•Post partum fatigue and depression

•Recurrent miscarriages, in particular in the path of 1st trimester

•Painful menstrual cramps or unexplained ignored periods

•Irregular menstrual cycle

•Ovarian cysts

•Uterine fibroids

•Endometriosis, and

•Premature menopause

Frequent Infections, Slow Healing

Examples encompass:

•Recurring urinary tract infections (UTI)

•Unexplained eye infections, and/or

•Slower than ordinary recuperation of even minor cuts and bruises

Mental or Emotional Signs

•Fuzzy questioning, thoughts fog or continual racing mind

•Irritability, specially underneath pressure

•Coping capability and feelings

•Can't interest or pay attention

•Feeling now not able to deal with strain

•Mild despair, and

•Feeling frazzled or scatter-brained

Miscellaneous Signs

•Hair loss

•Temperature intolerance (sensitivity to warmness and sunlight hours, cold arms and toes)

•Dry or upfront growing old pores and skin

•Chronic tinnitus (ringing within the ear)

•Dark circles under the eyes that don't disappear with relaxation

•Body aches and joint pain, and

•Muscle susceptible issue, loss of muscular tissues

Testing (or Lack There of)

Given the rift within the clinical community over whether or no longer or now not simply Adrenal Fatigue exists, I propose you to take terrific care as you discern to decide whether or not you clearly may also suffer from the syndrome.

Consult your clinical clinical doctor, however be prepared for him or her to tell you no longer anything is inaccurate. Listen for your intuition. If you KNOW a few issue is truely wrong with you, be geared up now not to permit your physician's loss of capability to assist get you down.

So, visit your scientific doctor, offer an motive of your symptoms and symptoms and signs, and ask for a stylish checkup and a complete blood test to make certain you don't produce other underlying nutrient deficiencies (which incorporates low nutrition B12, iron or nutrients D, to name just a few), hormonal imbalances or special fitness situations that need to be addressed.

If, after entire assessments had been finished, different motives have each been ruled out or addressed, and you continue to have the same signs and symptoms and symptoms, then you could keep in mind the cause of your symptoms and signs to be Adrenal Fatigue.

Unfortunately, your medical doctor or may not be inclined to refer you to all the recommended tests mentioned under because of the fact they're often no longer included with the useful resource of coverage. If this is the case, you may moreover paintings with an possibility health care practitioner with enjoy in Adrenal Fatigue (if feasible, as they will be tough to discover). Discuss all of your signs and signs and signs and symptoms and signs with them, what other clinical situations were identified and/or treated through your physician, and ask for a saliva check.

Ask to look the actual lab results, and then use the statistics underneath that will help you interpret the findings and stability that during opposition to what your medical doctor or practitioner is telling you.

Cortisol Tests

Cortisol may be measured thru urine, blood or saliva, and every clinical health practitioner may additionally have his or her desire. Many keep in mind saliva the maximum accurate technique, because it suggests cortisol stages at a mobile degree.

A single cortisol take a look at is not enough. Cortisol usually spikes inside the morning, dropping off over the route of the day. So, that lets in you to well decide the feature of your adrenal glands in producing cortisol, measurements taken at some of factors at some point of the day and mapped over a 24 hour length will tell your medical medical doctor plenty extra than a single test.

If you're seeing a health practitioner who doesn't have education or revel in, or doesn't keep in mind in Adrenal Fatigue, then the results are in all likelihood not going to be because it need to be interpreted. The laboratory's reference levels are often so massive that best the most intense consequences – at both the excessive or low quit – might be flagged.

What are the ones "everyday" stages? They will vary from laboratory to laboratory, and your scientific health practitioner, if he/she in all fairness modern-day, can also moreover make modifications to what he/she considers ordinary primarily based genuinely to your health and different elements.

As a elegant guide morning cortisol of 5 − 23 micrograms in keeping with deciliter (mcg/dL) within the morning or among three − 16 mcg/dL inside the afternoon may be taken into consideration "ordinary". The mission is that although consequences fall within this "normal" variety, this can now not simply rule out Adrenal Fatigue. It may be greater beneficial to observe "maximum beneficial" degrees, in place of "ordinary", or to take your effects to an opportunity medicinal drug practitioner with knowledge in Adrenal Fatigue.

ACTH

Once your baseline cortisol stages have been mapped, an ACTH (adrenal corticotrophin hormone) challenge check can be beneficial.

You may be injected with an ACTH dose, which mimics strain in stimulating your adrenal hormone production. Your cortisol tiers would be tested another time. As extended as there may be a marked spike, showing as approximately doubled for your blood check in comparison to the baseline cortisol take a look at, your adrenals are probable functioning properly. If the cortisol spike is much less than double, it suggests underperforming adrenals.

Thyroid

The thyroid additionally works on a feedback loop with the hypothalamus and pituitary glands, and this dating is known as the HPT axis. Remember that the adrenal glands are part of the HPA axis, and top-rated characteristic is interrelated. They're all part of the endocrine system. Any weakening of the pituitary or hypothalamus glands, which takes location in Adrenal Fatigue, can bring about lower thyroid function. The mission is that the equal antique stages for "ordinary" utilized by labs and the doctors who interpret the tests don't correctly endure in mind the nuances of hypothyroidism, nor the reality that hypothyroidism itself may be because of Adrenal Fatigue.

TSH

The pituitary gland produces thyroid-stimulating hormone (TSH), which in turn turns on the thyroid to generate T3 and T4. If your thyroid gland is luckily churning out good enough quantities of T3 and T4, your TSH degrees can be lower due to the fact the thyroid doesn't want as lots stimulation. On the alternative hand, if your T3 and T4 levels are lower, indicating you're hypothyroid, then your TSH will probable be higher, because your hypothalamus is sending more thyroid stimulating hormone, telling your thyroid it wants to offer more of the essential T3 and T4 hormones.

The laboratory reference stages for "regular" TSH range barely lab to lab, however normally fall in the zero.Four – four.Zero gadgets per milliliter variety. Those stricken by Adrenal Fatigue frequently have poorly appearing thyroid glands and the TSH level might be above 2.Zero. Perhaps now not enough to prompt your scientific medical doctor to reserve treatment, but, combined with specific tests, also can moreover assist you and your alternative medication professional to attain a assessment of Adrenal Fatigue.

T3 and T4

T4 is extra adequate in the bloodstream, however T3 is clearly responsible for maximum of the frame's metabolic hobby. Both T3 and T4 are constituted of free, or "unbound", hormones which is probably to be had for your tissues and cells to use proper away, alongside element hormone this is "positive" to protein cells. The Free T3 and T4 is the maximum beneficial size because it gives a clearer picture to diagnosticians. For favored T4, the ordinary range for adults is ready five to 14 mcg/dL (micrograms in keeping with deciliter), even as loose T4's normal range is prepared zero.Eight – hundred ng/dL (nanograms everyday with deciliter). For total T3, search for effects between approximately 80 and hundred ng/dL and a couple of.Three – 4.2 pg/dL (pictograms constant with deciliter) with out price T3.

Side Note: If you believe you studied you have a thyroid hassle but the above thyroid checks are within "regular" lab degrees consistent with your scientific health practitioner, keep in mind having a complete thyroid panel check completed, which incorporates TSH, Free T4, Free T3, Reverse T3, and Thyroid Antibodies. However, all of those tests are regularly NOT finished through medical doctors as they will rely upon TSH on my own, which does now not offer a complete observe of thyroid feature. You may additionally furthermore pick out to go to a modern thyroid professional or possibility healthcare practitioner alternatively. Iodine deficiency can also motive adrenal and thyroid symptoms and signs and symptoms. If you decided you have iodine deficiency, artwork with a expert to behavior finding out and administer iodine supplementation (it is a touchy method that requires tailor-made guidance from a knowledgeable, iodine-aware practitioner).

Blood Pressure Test

Comparing results of blood strain assessments among sitting and standing positions can show functionality Adrenal Fatigue. The first studying need to be taken once you've been resting for about five mins and are pretty comfortable. Then get up right away, and take your blood stress another time.

Chapter 5: Curing Adrenal Fatigue Naturally:

Diet, Vitamins & Supplements

When you're under stress, your body needs extra nutritious gas than it'd in any other case. The key right right here is nutritious. Fast meals actually ain't it. Along with what you consume, on the same time as you eat is likewise important. Eating regularly – and eating sufficient – allows keep cortisol ranges stable so the adrenal glands don't want to art work quite so tough. The answer is to take within the right gasoline and reduce ability dietary stressors to make sure our our bodies run easily and optimally, which as a end result, will beneficial useful resource in recuperation Adrenal Fatigue.

Based on my own personal recuperation revel in with Adrenal Fatigue, plus many success recollections of actual human beings, I truely have with out cease researched the outcomes of weight loss plan in healing the human body – and the solution seems so simple. In curing Adrenal Fatigue, selected a food regimen that is easy, entire, and comes from nature; along with plant-primarily based surely, immoderate nutrient entire food. Eating a diet rich in plant-based totally absolutely food is established to lower the general hazard of ailment and places masses much less stress on our adrenal glands, which I will deal with in extra detail within the direction of this financial ruin.

Though this can not be renowned as a 'conventional' technique in a society complete of advertising and advertising and marketing, fad diets and falsity, there are various knowledgeable, noticeably knowledgeable, and well-respectable scientific scientific medical docs who percent this view (and from whom I truly have discovered out), who have successfully helped their sufferers emerge as well once more. You might also furthermore locate different opposing techniques to be had that claim to remedy Adrenal Fatigue, to which I disagree – I honestly have attempted the ones suggestions and discovered they made my signs and symptoms worse and did no longer artwork for me within the long-time period.

Dr. Neal Barnard has written considerably about stopping most cancers with a plant-based totally absolutely healthy dietweight-reduction plan. He references records that suggests the risk of demise from maximum cancers will boom among 14 and 50 percentage for individuals who frequently devour crimson and processed meats and who devour excessive-fats dairy. Dr. Dean Ornish, Dr. John McDougall, Dr. Joel Fuhrman and Dr. Caldwell Esselstyn also are proactive nutrients specialists, each selling a weight-reduction plan that is plant-based totally honestly and low in fat to prevent, or opposite, coronary heart disease and high-quality illnesses. If you do your very non-public studies, as I actually have, you'll discover other examples of scientific clinical doctors who've 'visible the mild' and are promoting the electricity of desire in healthy eating plan and manner of existence in reversing or stopping contamination and dramatically enhancing how we revel in. Adrenal Fatigue is one of the syndromes that may be reversed with a chunk schooling and attempt, and it's my satisfaction to help you along your journey.

Diet

Choose the Right Foods

Plant-Based Foods

A plant-based totally absolutely in reality weight-reduction plan is focused on veggies, quit result, entire grains (ideally gluten loose varieties for adrenal recovery), legumes, nuts and seeds, with very little animal products. Some examples may also encompass cucumbers, apples, leafy veggies, broccoli, mushrooms, brown rice, berries, beans, lentils and peas, simply to call a few. Colorful plant substances encompass herbal phytochemicals, fiber and antioxidants (which assist shield our our bodies from contamination and allows our commonplace health), and gives our our bodies with plentiful vitamins which includes iron and calcium. Though ingesting one hundred percent plant-based is good, if you are transitioning, I do encourage you try to have at the least eighty five percent of your food plan (the greater the higher) made up of those nutrient-dense, non-processed food for quicker healing. You will look at how a splendid deal higher you begin to experience proper away.

Whole Foods

The opposite of processed. It definitely method being attentive to consuming meals that looks as near what it did at the same time as it became growing in nature, with the least amount of processing feasible. Not that each one processing is lousy, both. The processing you do to your non-public kitchen, say making applesauce from natural apples, is nice and needn't be averted. Ready-made elements or condiments that include simple, herbal, plant-based components are also a fantastic addition in your complete food food – you could discover ways to have a look at labels like a pro.

The Carb Conundrum

Carbohydrates are the macronutrient our our our bodies require within the most vital portions, as they are our vital deliver of electricity and gas for our bodies (and our minds!) to feature optimally – an critical key in stopping low moods and strength stages in Adrenal Fatigue.

Many processed carbohydrate elements are taken into consideration 'smooth carbs', that might metabolize fast and come to be brief bursts of strength highs and lows. Examples of processed clean carbs encompass white desk sugar, observed in jams and jellies, easy drinks or sweets, which incorporate little nutritional benefit. Avoid those processed carbs and choose whole meals containing natural, easy sugars (like fruit), that are higher metabolized via the frame with its fiber, proteins, nutrients and minerals in spite of the fact that during tact.

Many human beings fear fruit underneath the guise that it is the handiest perpetrator for blood sugar spikes. This, however, is wrong and depends how the sugars are harmonized with more fats in the diet regime (specially saturated fats), which I will cope with within the following section. During the initial degrees of your restoration at the same time as your body is adjusting to its new weight loss program, it's nice to consume surrender end result and smooth juices earlier inside the day, and as your Adrenal Fatigue stabilizes you can preserve to comprise more fruits into your weight loss plan to revel in in abundance.

'Complex carbs' also are complete of fiber, vitamins and minerals. They are fulfilling as they take longer to digest, are used by the frame for lengthy-time period electricity launch, and might truly accelerate your metabolism in order that your body burns energy extra correctly. Examples encompass whole plant meals like starchy greens (potatoes, candy potatoes, yams, pumpkin and corn), and complete grains (ideally gluten loose) – opt for brown rice over white rice, in particular at a few stage inside the first segment of recovery. These are all exceptional options to include in your healthy dietweight-reduction plan at any time of day.

Don't Avoid Carbs

It's regarding to look such quite a few women and men cut carbohydrates out in their weight loss plan inside the hopes they'll shed pounds, at the same time as in truth, it can have quite the possibility bring about the extended-time period. Avoiding carbs is a commonplace mistake and might make Adrenal Fatigue worse, and proper right here's why.

We've cited the relationship amongst hypothyroidism and Adrenal Fatigue. Carbs without delay have an impact on thyroid function. Carbohydrates get transformed into the glucose (sugar), which suits together with insulin to provide electricity. Insulin is needed to convert T4 (the inactive hormone) into T3 (the active hormone). Low carbs = low insulin = low thyroid and increased signs and symptoms and signs, which embody extended-time period weight gain.

Cortisol, the principle hormone produced with the resource of the adrenal glands, has a tendency to boom even as on a low carb food plan because of the reality the frame wants to stability out its glucose levels. This approach it's far a functionality stressor in your adrenal device. If you're already affected by Adrenal Fatigue Syndrome, or are prone and suspect you may have AFS, together with a low carb diet plan to a traumatic method, horrific sleep and possibly immoderate exercising, and voila. You've simply perfected the recipe for burnout!

Excess fats in the blood (specially from animal merchandise and processed oils) obstructs the delivery of glucose to our cells for electricity, which overworks our adrenals, creates an adrenalin rush, and outcomes in a blood sugar spike or insulin resistance. Some people want to address this hassle with the aid of casting off carbohydrates from their diet plan. You have to expect this may make sense, right? But this shows most in their eating regimen can be crafted from fats and protein – and as we recognize through now, a whole host of fitness issues can happen if the frame is missing an essential deliver of gas to characteristic well.

Maintaining strong glucose stages will offer you with maximum suitable fat burning standard performance, increase your electricity degrees, have a wonderful effect in your mood and control your urge for food at the equal time as minimizing food cravings. So, don't be terrified of complex carbohydrates and herbal sugars in plant-primarily based whole food.

Limit Gluten Grains and Concentrated Sugar

These culprits can also contribute to impaired insulin response, HPA disease and stylish inflammation. Lara Briden, a Canadian-knowledgeable Naturopathic Doctor now certified and training in Australia, calls gluten grains and focused sugar "un-mild carbs", and promotes avoidance for people with hormone imbalance problems like Adrenal Fatigue.

But Briden and other specialists do endorse intake of "mild carbs", which can be the carbs that do not promote contamination.

Root vegetables like beet, potato and candy potato, and entire grains like brown rice, quinoa, buckwheat, millet or amaranth are outstanding complex carbohydrates to feed an adrenal fatigued frame. Eating moderate quantities is usually recommended as beneficial in helping adrenal characteristic.

It is also very crucial to discover and cast off each other food that you are allergic or illiberal to. Food sensitivities are very common and can be worsening your symptoms and symptoms and signs. Common offenders embody wheat, gluten, dairy, eggs, soy and plenty of others.

What About Protein?

Proteins are placed in all elements (even in give up quit result and greens) in sufficient quantities for our bodies to thrive. For the initial remedy of Adrenal Fatigue no matter the fact that, it is advocated to often eat a small part of protein wealthy food (plant-based, of path, like beans, nuts, seeds, or legumes) alongside side your moderate, slow carbs. This will result in even higher blood sugar balance – powerful for those humans with insulin sensitivities, that is available in hand with having Adrenal Fatigue. If you pick to eat soy products (high-quality cautiously in case you aren't intolerant or sensitive), select herbal soy with the least processing viable, which includes tempeh or organic tofu.

There are numerous critiques concerning every day macronutrient ratios – what labored for me for the duration of my recovery way end up a diploma of about 60% carbohydrates, 25% protein and 15% fat. Rather than being meticulous with this, I recommend which you surely make certain fat does not exceed about 20 to 20-five% of your each day intake, and make certain you're consuming more proper carbohydrates than proteins to preserve sufficient power ranges. Everyone's protocol is probably barely particular, as each person's metabolic price and united states of america of health is one-of-a-type. The common emphasis is on entire meals, so you may additionally moreover moreover check a touch with ratios to sense what works fantastic in your body and what's going to first-rate can help you stick with a whole meals weight loss program. As your frame adjusts to its new diet plan, begins offevolved offevolved to heal and balances its insulin, you could slowly growth your carbohydrate ratio to in that you revel in maximum happy.

Facts About Fat

Fats are an essential part of our eating regimen, but it's miles the terrific and amount of fat that we need to be conscious of. We frequently pay attention approximately the blessings of a Mediterranean weight loss plan and prefer to characteristic this to using olive oil, however what is regularly unnoticed is the overall nutritional pattern – a menu wealthy in unrefined plant meals with a completely confined consumption of dairy and meat.

What has worked efficaciously for plenty people who have suffered from Adrenal Fatigue is getting rid of saturated fat (usually discovered in animal products) and proscribing processed oils, yet even though playing the whole food version moderately to accumulate complete nutritional advantage (i.E. Whole olives in place of olive oil, coconut meat in region of coconut oil, avocado over avocado oil, whole nuts and seeds over nut oils).

According to Dr. John McDougall, "our our our bodies can synthesize most fats from carbohydrates and there are only some unsaturated fats that our our bodies can't make with the useful resource of way of themselves". As a end result, there can be no want to overload our our our our bodies with greater fats and processed oils, that can overwork our pancreas and forces our adrenal glands to provide more adrenaline (which over time, can bring about a mess of fitness issues because of awful weight loss program, which incorporates Adrenal Fatigue).

Contrary to diverse reviews, processed oils, which include vegetable oils, olive or perhaps coconut oil, aren't healthy specially for those suffering from Adrenal Fatigue. Hydrogenated oils, even though they sound like they arrive from a healthful supply, like soybean, corn or canola, have a tendency to be very inflammatory and may stimulate your adrenal glands – and even as heated end up rancid and carcinogenic. Oils are also calorie dense whilst thinking about their low nutrient fee, as they may be stripped of fiber, making them effortlessly absorbed into the bloodstream – a recipe for easy fat storage.

Minimizing oils can be a task at the begin, so attempt cooking with vegetable broths, organic soy sauce (tamari), tomato juice or a sprint of water while sautéing in a non-stick frying pan. In baking, you can update oil with food like applesauce or mashed bananas to characteristic texture and moisture.

Calorie Restriction? Never.

Unfortunately, our preference for instant and speedy outcomes can regularly negatively have an effect on our health. Crash diets and calorie restrict might also get you for your purpose weight 'faster' in the quick-time period, however ask your self, will you be able to keep the identical nutritional conduct for all time? Will you keep the burden off? And will this damage your health and your metabolism inside the prolonged-time period? You WILL be capable of get to a wholesome weight and maintain it as speedy as you have healed your frame and usually eat healthfully. Patience and consistency is fundamental.

It's simply critical not to beneath consume. Not ingesting enough or going lengthy durations without a nutritious snack can positioned your frame into extra stress. It thinks there can be starvation on the horizon and is going into protection mode (have a observe: stress), setting more desires in your already-worn-out adrenals. Don't starve your cells of herbal electricity with the beneficial aid of keeping off or severely proscribing food – make certain to preserve your frame fuelled inside the route of the day and NEVER bypass breakfast. This isn't a allow to stuff your self, even though – in reality honor your starvation and absolutely located down the fork whilst you are glad.

You will discover that on a plant-based clearly diet regime, you can need to devour quite a piece more in quantity than you is probably used to as a manner to get in enough energy for optimum adrenal feature – that is because of the fact plant additives are complete of fiber and water, even as processed substances are frequently encompass centered 'empty electricity' laden with processed oil and diffused sugar. A wholesome bean salad also can comprise lesser energy than a small, greasy pastry, as an instance. Every man or woman's consumption can be excellent, however try and goal for at the least the identical quantity of electricity which you were eating preceding to switching to finish elements, or maybe greater if you have been proscribing.

When you first begin removing addictive, processed meals out of your diet plan, you could find out you continue to having cravings for them in the beginning. Whilst you're suffering with these cravings, don't be afraid to load up your plate with wholesome plant ingredients, and snack frequently. The greater happy you are, the lots less possibilities you will obtain for that bag of chips!

Sweets and Treats

If you find you're yearning goodies, as severa us with Adrenal Fatigue do, select entire food with natural sugars collectively with entire end result. Instead of touchy white sugar, you can replace with extra wholesome sweeteners carefully (reduce at a few stage in the early tiers of your restoration approach), which incorporates coconut sugar, herbal maple syrup, stevia, dates or herbal date syrup. Avoid using synthetic chemical sweeteners, which can wreak havoc for your fitness and metabolism.

Also pay interest that a few cereals, breads, dressings and condiments can regularly incorporate white sugar, every now and then in relatively massive quantities, so make sure to test labels and select merchandise with wholesome elements. Choose excessive high-quality bread made with complete grains (gluten free is tremendous), in choice to processed, white flour. Opt for gluten unfastened herbal oats, puffed brown rice or quinoa flakes, as an instance, topped with smooth cease result and seeds in vicinity of extraordinarily processed cereals containing sugar.

Salt Surprise

Healthy adrenal characteristic requires sodium, and sodium is generally low in the ones suffering Adrenal Fatigue. Unless you're an individual with Adrenal Fatigue and excessive blood pressure, it's not a remarkable idea to restriction your salt intake. Be high quality not to overdo it each – a pinch or introduced to meals is adequate, and pick out out immoderate super sea salt. Celtic or Himalayan sea salt are outstanding alternatives due to the fact further they incorporate certainly one of a type important minerals and nutrients that the processing of traditional desk salt has eliminated.

Ditch the Dairy

Commercial dairy merchandise are pasteurized, which makes the protein within the dairy product extra hard to digest. This results in more infection in the frame. How does the body respond to extended contamination? The adrenal glands produce cortisol. Bingo. Avoiding dairy products lets in reduce infection, which permits the adrenal glands cling directly to its cortisol.

According to Dr. Michael Greger (physician and across the world identified fitness and nutrients speaker), the consumption of dairy products has moreover been linked to various hormonal imbalances, pimples, immoderate ldl ldl cholesterol, most cancers, coronary coronary heart sickness and diabetes, really to name some − yep, even diabetes. We are often misinformed that sugar (even from herbal sources) is the purpose of insulin problems, whilst in fact, a further of saturated fat placed in animal merchandise (dairy, eggs and meat) creates more acidity inside the body, reducing its ability to regulate insulin stages. This is a bad facts for anyone, especially the ones parents with Adrenal Fatigue with already hindered insulin law. Why located your health at risk? Reduce your consumption of animal merchandise and make the smooth transfer over to natural milk options, like almond, rice or coconut, if you're searching for a milk-kind beverage.

Go Organic

Many with Adrenal Fatigue Syndrome cannot tolerate the insecticides, herbicides, antibiotics or extraordinary chemical compounds sprayed onto or fed into our food as it's far grown or produced. Eating natural produce everywhere possible permits lessen our toxic load. Consuming natural ocean veggies, like seaweed, helps to offer trace iodine, which supports thyroid function.

Stay Hydrated

Fluid "dis-regulation" is a commonplace problem in Adrenal Fatigue. The adrenalin launched while the frame is underneath pressure will increase the fee of urine float, and consistent with Dr. Michael Lam, most Adrenal Fatigue sufferers are in a few level of fluid depletion or dehydration.

Make fantastic you're eating enough spring or filtered water (a higher opportunity than tap water which may be chlorinated and fluoridated in lots of municipal water structures) to assist your body maintain fluid balance. As a extensive guide, you should attempt to drink an ounces. Of water for each pound you weigh, consistent with day (about 33ml normal with kilogram).

Additionally, ingesting sparkling coconut water (commonly known as "nature's Gatorade") additionally works effectively in hydrating and replenishing electrolytes.

Steer Clear of Stimulants

Omit stimulants together with caffeine, cacao, energy beverages, tablets, and alcohol. The brief-time period enhance you experience is destructive for your healing. They spark off your adrenals to make cortisol and adrenalin, mimicking the 'fight or flight' strain reaction, that is clearly such as to the weight for your tired adrenals. Try changing cacao (or cocoa) with powdered carob if growing your personal wholesome treats. Carob makes a wonderful stimulant-free possibility for the honest chocoholic.

Green tea is appropriate sparsely, which you could drink in substitute of your normal cup of espresso to assist ditch the dependancy and cut caffeine cravings. It should be seemed that coffee is likewise a diuretic, that means it gets rid of water out of your body causing dehydration. Coffee is likewise acidic, and can be worrying to the belly and disillusioned digestion, and as a stimulant can maintain you unsleeping at night time time (to the detriment in your adrenals).

Teas Between Meals

Another brilliant manner to hydrate and provide your body with vitamins, specifically amongst meals, is to brew and drink caffeine unfastened, entire leaf, herbal herbal teas. Not black tea, because of its caffeine content material cloth, but teas with immoderate antioxidant and anti inflammatory functions. Some brilliant teas for adrenal assist embody licorice tea, hibiscus (flor de Jamaica), that is full of antioxidants and vitamins C, and rooibos (or pink tea), which has been studied to ease the symptoms of stress and lower stress hormone levels. Coldwater steeping can also result in better concentrations of nutrients than warm steeping, in particular for hibiscus tea. Dandelion tea is also full of vitamins and minerals, and dandelion 'espresso' is a awesome substitute for folks that are lacking the wealthy taste in their ordinary espresso repair. Consume teas with warning in case you are pregnant.

Timing of Meals

Eating hastily after you've got up is one of the maximum crucial changes you can make in addressing your Adrenal Fatigue. Overnight, your blood sugar stages drop, and the longer you wait inside the morning to devour a nutritious breakfast, the bigger the choice for you are placing to your adrenals to pressure your body without food. Breakfast internal half of-hour of waking is proper. If you may't stomach that, breakfast ought to be consumed in the hour.

An early lunch is also vital, due to the truth your frame will burn thru its breakfast quite brief. The excellent time for lunch is among 11:30am and 12pm. Also purpose for a stable snack among 2 and 3 pm that will help you adventure via the cortisol low that we recognize is coming among three and four.

Aim for a dinner party among 5 and six pm, and plan for a immoderate exquisite snack approximately 30-forty five minutes earlier than bed to help you weather sleep disturbances. (I will communicate greater about sleep inside the subsequent bankruptcy.)

Snacking

Those stricken by Adrenal Fatigue frequently have hassle preserving blood sugar stages. Yes, your blood test results can also display regular, but you can nonetheless display off signs and symptoms of hypoglycemia: dizziness, tension, fatigue, and occasionally even a revel in of being drowned. Healthy commonplace snacking is one of the exquisite processes to remove those signs and symptoms and signs. Get into the dependancy of sporting a snack with you anyplace you cross. Taking a nutritious snack truely earlier than bed may assist you go to sleep simpler, and live asleep, due to the fact your blood sugar is in higher stability. Here are a few healthful Adrenal Fatigue snacking hints:

•Slightly salted snacks are useful, as people with Adrenal Fatigue Syndrome are regularly in a salt depletion nation because of the aldosterone dysregulation.

•Nuts – natural and uncooked tree nuts, like almonds, walnuts, cashews, pistachios, macadamias or pecans. Peanuts are not simply nuts, they're from the legume own family, and in addition to being a not unusual allergen they can also motive inner inflammation. Sorry peanut butter fans, no peanuts in the route of the initial tiers of your restoration manner.

•Organic and uncooked route blend.

•Fresh stop end result which incorporates apples, pears, berries, cherries, mango, stone fruit or bananas to preserve strength stages.

•Organic dried give up end result, as soon as your Adrenal Fatigue is stabilized, which incorporates goji berries, cranberries, blueberries, mulberries and goldenberries.

•Plain, unbuttered popcorn with sea salt.

•Hummus (made with natural tahini) and smooth vegetables like carrots, celery or bell peppers.

•Wholegrain crackers (can be made from brown rice, corn or quinoa) topped with avocado, tomato, radish, sea salt and pepper.

Help Heal the Adrenals with These Foods

•Seaweeds (kelp, wakame, nori, kombu, dulse)

•Sprouts and leafy greens

•Whole food carbohydrates

•Whole fat reasonably, which encompass avocado and coconut

- Berries

- Carob

- Sea salt

- Miso, fermented manifestly without MSG

- Red and orange vegetables

- Cruciferous vegetables, broccoli, cauliflower, kale

- Vegetable juices

- Ginger

- Almonds, chia seeds and flaxseeds

- Beans and legumes, whilst blended with wholegrain food, and

- Licorice tea.

Avoid Foods that Hurt Adrenals

- Coffee and black tea

- Refined sugars

•Alcohol

•Deep-fried anything

•Processed food

•Saturated fats, together with meat, cheese and eggs

•Addictive fast food and junk meals

•Any food to which you are touchy or allergic

•Milk and dairy products

•Products containing fantastically subtle flours (pasta, bread, cookies, pies, desserts, and so on)

•Gluten (restriction wherein viable or dispose of if you are touchy)

•Chocolate (containing cacao, cocoa, dairy or sugar)

•Rancid oils, nuts and seeds (even 'proper' oils pass horrible, frequently rapid), and

•Artificial sweeteners, artificial components.

Supplements and Herbal Support

Common mistakes in Adrenal Fatigue recovery embody the use of dietary dietary dietary supplements and prescription medicines improperly, regularly taking too much that could upload extra stress on the body. Vitamin dietary supplements and herbal drug treatments need to handiest be applied in concert with the hints on this e-book for a healthful, balanced weight loss program, and never as a substitute for wholesome ingesting.

It is also essential to preserve in mind that nutritional dietary dietary supplements are not regulated, and there are unethical manufacturers reachable who're more interested by income quantity and earnings than your well being. As nicely, loss of investment for research into capacity toxic effects way there's little to no "famous dosage" facts. And, how one character responds to 1 dose of a nutritional or natural supplement can be quite wonderful from each other.

Okay, now permit's test some of the nutrients and herbs which have assisted many humans in improving from Adrenal Fatigue. You can benefit the numerous nutrients and minerals said from herbal food sources, despite the fact that a few extra supplementation may additionally moreover assist pork up your recuperation technique.

Herbal Remedies

Herbal remedy is older than civilization. Animals of a wide range will deliberately devour unique flowers as a way to address viruses, micro organism, worms or parasites. History tells us that Aboriginal and Chinese healers going decrease returned millennia have regarded to the vegetation provided thru Mother Nature to heal and preserve the frame in stability.

Here are a number of the most common, and effective, herbs that are useful in addressing Adrenal Fatigue.

 Licorice Root (Glycyrrhizin Glabra and G. Uralensis)

Licorice is drastically used to deal with Adrenal Insufficiency further to ulcers. It permits effect the stability of cortisone and cortisol inside the body. Adrenal blessings can be determined with just small doses of licorice, about 25 – seventy five mg of standardized extract per day. Available in tablet or liquid extract shape, licorice use is stated to have superior health advantages inside the areas of blood sugar control, better absorption of iron, reduced infection, progressed hormone stability in girls, and recovery of the liner of the gut. (Note that licorice is not related to anise, big call anise, or fennel, irrespective of the taste similarities. When looking for a licorice herbal complement, make certain you have become the actual element and not a product made with the less costly anise.)

Ginkgo Leaf (Ginkgo Biloba)

It is commonly recognised that Ginkgo helps beautify skip, however it could honestly have a beneficial impact on stress tiers. For heaps of years, the Chinese have notably applied Ginkgo for a number of troubles from asthma and libido assist to anti-growing old. Ginkgo is also connected to beneficial mind characteristic outcomes like stepped forward alertness and reminiscence, and decreased mind fog and highbrow fatigue. Ginkgo specially permits with Adrenal Fatigue via its anti-oxidative houses, which help shield the adrenals from capability unfastened radical damage.

Again, not all Ginkgo products are the same first-rate. Look for standardized extracts with 24 percentage ginkgo flavones and glycosides, and 6 percent bilobalides and ginkgolides. Ginkgo is likewise to be had in liquid or tablet form.

Korean Ginseng Root (Panax Ginseng)

Western natural treatment practitioners use the precept root of the Korean Ginseng plant to cope with bodily or highbrow exhaustion. However, in traditional Chinese medicinal drug it is used to promote sturdiness and improve critical electricity. Recent research have supported using Korean Ginseng root to help with insulin sensitivity, higher blood flow in the mind, stepped forward immune system and treatment from some signs of menopause. If you've got troubles with sleep disturbances, it isn't always encouraged that you take Panax Ginseng any later than noon.

Siberian Ginseng Root (Eleutherococus Senticosus)

Sometimes called Eleuthero, this herb allows with intellectual processing, immune function and stress. What's in reality taking region is that the Siberian Ginseng Root acts like a slight stressor to the frame, and it's the frame's very very own reaction to the stress that money owed for the referred to therapeutic advantages. For this cause, satisfactory human beings with mild Adrenal Fatigue should use this herb short time period to avoid overwhelming the frame's strain reaction tool similarly and demanding the situation over time.

Ashwagandha (Withania Somnifera)

This is an historic Indian herb that has been widely used by India's Ayurvedic physicians for a number of healing features, which consist of advanced feature of the adrenal glands. Ashwagandha is a substance that enables the frame return to everyday. If cortisol is definitely too excessive, taking Ashwagandha will help decrease it. If cortisol is clearly too low, Ashwagandha will help increase it. Taking Ashwagandha right in advance than bedtime can assist enhance the notable of sleep for some human beings.

Ginger Root (Zingiber Officinale)

Ginger root permits deliver blood strain and heart charge decrease lower back into regular stages, ends in extended strength and metabolic fee, which in flip allows to burn fat. It is likewise stated to stimulate digestive enzyme secretions that assist the frame soak up proteins and fatty acids.

Those with diabetes, liver infection or alcohol dependence have to use caution the use of ginger root. Liquid preparations of ginger root frequently consist of alcohol and/or sugar. In some arrangements, ginger root also includes aristolochic acid, which can also bring about kidney or urinary gadget sickness. Signs encompass blood within the urine or an uncommon trade in the quantity of urine produced. Pregnant or breast-feeding ladies have to moreover avoid the use of ginger root products.

A Note About Stimulating Effects

If you word progressed energy and lots a lot less fatigue at the same time as taking any of the above herbal dietary dietary dietary supplements, you'll be tempted to have fun. However, as referred to via Dr. Michael Lam, the extra mentioned you sense this stimulation, the greater immoderate your Adrenal Fatigue, and you can really be in addition depleting your adrenals as they artwork extra difficult to keep the stimulated state. If you experience essential stimulation or every other unusual thing impact you need to reduce all over again and modify your quantities.

Vitamins and Minerals

There are some of diet and mineral dietary supplements that can help guide adrenal function. Not all of these listed nutritional supplements might be appropriate or essential for every person, so you can also additionally moreover pick out to eat them through gentle food sources instead. The consequences of your saliva and certainly one of a kind exams will assist you and your medical doctor, if you have one, determine which of these dietary dietary supplements can be right for you.

Vitamin C

Vitamin C is one of the key nutrients that can substantially help recovery from Adrenal Fatigue. It's an antioxidant that works directly with the adrenals to deliver cortisol. Vitamin C additionally enhances absorption of iron to assist combat anemia. In addition, it's well known to assist beautify the immune device and protect in competition to loose radicals. 1000mcg is a great starting dose. Look for liposomal or buffered weight loss plan C.

Food property: Raspberries, sprouts, papaya, kiwi, inexperienced leafy vegetables, tomatoes, hibiscus tea, citrus stop cease result, strawberries, amla (gooseberry) powder, citrus fruit, broccoli, purple or yellow bell peppers.

B Vitamins

B12, B6 and B5 all make contributions to mobile metabolic function. Taking immoderate incredible B dietary supplements can assist enhance electricity. Specifically, B12 allows with cellular restore and purple blood mobile protection; B6 allows create adrenal hormones; B5 allows harm down proteins, carbs and fat. Aim for baseline doses of one hundred mcg of B12, 50mg of B6, and 1000mg of B5.

Food resources: Nutritional yeast, brewers yeast, nuts, miso, whole grains, potato, avocado, soybeans (and edamame), bananas, lentils.

Magnesium

Studies suggest that as many as 75 percent of Americans are magnesium bad, with produces symptoms of fatigue, depression, insomnia and muscle cramping. Too lots magnesium can produce digestive problems, so start with a four hundred mg dose to make certain you could tolerate it.

Food sources: Sesame seeds (or tahini), quinoa, pumpkin seeds, kidney beans, spinach, almonds, tempeh, green greens, wild rice, dates, flaxseed.

Selenium

Selenium is an crucial hint mineral this is critical for healthy thyroid and adrenal function and moreover protects from cellular damage. Ingesting too much selenium can be toxic, so in case you pick to take a supplement, attempt no extra than two hundred mcg each couple of days, briefly, in a few unspecified time within the future of your recuperation manner.

Food resources: Mustard, brown rice, brazil nuts, cabbage, chia seeds, arrowroot powder, mushrooms, onions, sunflower seeds.

Probiotics

Probiotics help improve digestion, which permits the frame approach more of the vitamins in our meals. They additionally offer immune device aid. Look for a dairy unfastened probiotic complement that has at least 5 lines of bacteria, together with Lactobacillus acidophilus DDS-1, and 10 billion CFUs (colony forming devices).

Food sources: Sauerkraut, kimchi, kombucha tea, miso, pickles, olives, nut milks.

Other Helpful Supplements

These compounds may be useful and are all with out troubles to be had on-line and at maximum pharmacies or fitness meals stores. Try Omega-3 (non-fish and plant-derived) to help lessen infection, CoQ10 to supply energy and keep cell feature, Acetyl-L-Carnitine to reinforce metabolism, and a plant-derived Vitamin D complement in case you are not soaking up at least 15 minutes of sunlight hours every day.

Chapter 6: Curing Adrenal Fatigue Naturally:

Sleep, Rest & Exercise

Sleep, relaxation and exercise all play key roles in dealing with and recovering from pressure. Even exercising – normally touted as a obligatory element in suitable fitness – can reason extra stress if now not done correctly for your person degree of adrenal health. Falling via the cracks amongst sleep and exercise is rest. Simple rest. I consider that each one three need to take shipping of same priority on your adrenal fatigue healing plan.

Sleep and Sleep Hygiene

How is your sleep? The significance of doing all you can to make sure you get adequate, restful and restorative sleep can't be overstated. Too hundreds of us have allow sleep take the backseat to specific existence priorities. We have superior bedtime conduct that get in the manner of proper and restful sleep. Whether the stop end result is Adrenal Fatigue, or genuinely perpetual exhaustion, being attentive to sleep hygiene could make a extensive distinction.

 What is Sleep Hygiene?

Sleep hygiene is a term used to explain some of practices that help make sure that midnight is whole of amazing sleep, and daylight is complete of alertness. The most important of all the practices is to set up a everyday, 7-day-in line with-week, sleep and wake pattern. Not a Monday-Friday pattern, and each different for the weekends. This consists of spending the proper amount of time in mattress. Here is a list of endorsed and wholesome sleep hygiene practices:

•Discipline your self to order your mattress for the two "s" sports activities sports, sex and sleep. Avoid looking TV, running for your computer, or even studying.

•Eliminate caffeine, nicotine and alcohol. Alcohol may additionally moreover help you get to sleep, but as your body begins to metabolize the alcohol it wakes you up and disrupts your sleep.

•Exercise: full of life workout is k in the morning or afternoon, IF this doesn't purpose an adrenal crash, however limit evening workout to amusing kinds of hobby like yoga (I'll get into workout in extra element fast).

•Make positive you get enough natural mild. If you have got were given been cooped up indoors, whether or not due to iciness or infection, find out a manner to show your self to 3 sunshine – the 'satisfied' nutrients. This moreover lets in the frame understand the distinction between day and night and beef up the message that sunlight hours is for waking and middle of the night for sleep.

•No daylight sleeping. It can disrupt the vital circadian rhythm of the sleep-massive extensive wakeful cycles.

•Don't eat too near bedtime, and recollect that any changes in your food regimen may also additionally cause sleep troubles.

•Set up a bedtime recurring that is fun. Avoid emotionally horrifying conversations simply earlier than you could sleep.

•Restrict the use of electronics within the half of hour before bed and eliminate them in mattress. The moderate from the incredible video display units works to trick your thoughts into wondering it's miles daytime. At the very least, located your show display on the dimmest possible putting if you need to apply the tool inside the middle of the night hours important to bedtime.

Rest, Relax and Reduce Stress

Rest, relaxation and then rest some extra. Once you've finished that, discover a suitable spot to sit down down or lie down, and relaxation. Okay, I jest. But best a little.

Examine the way you have been engaging in your existence, and be aware how generally in the course of a day you "push on through" because of the fact you think you want to "get subjects executed". This is conduct that has contributed in your scenario, and you need to prevent. Taking a five-minute harm among responsibilities isn't always going to make a large dent on your productiveness, however it's far going that will help you reclaim your fitness.

Managing Stress

Stress is frequently considered as some component that happens "to" us, some thing this is past our manipulate. With that mindset, we're sufferers, powerless to alternate how strain affects us. If this resonates with you, and sounds right for you, I actually have records.

You do have the power to select out your response to the outside event. Mindfulness physical games can be very beneficial in education the manner to split the "judgments" we follow to nearly every situation, idea, movement, and procedure in our lives from the subjects themselves. This allows to lessen the emotional responses, regularly disturbing, and lets in us to view topics greater objectively.

Worrying is an instance. Decide to have a outstanding mind-set and frequently a listing of concerns shrinks extensively. Ask yourself if the difficulty is a few issue internal your manage, or outside your manage? If it's a few factor that is beyond your control, bypass it off the listing. Worrying is harming your health. If it in fact is a choice you need to make, strive growing a notice of it or write about it in a journal, and located it away for over again. But no longer absolutely before bed, wherein it's going to intervene in conjunction with your sleep.

Look for strategies to shift your views and attitudes on life, as critical. Examples encompass training gratitude, appreciation, letting skip, forgiveness, and exploring spirituality. All of these are effective adjustments that produce terrific trade in how your frame and mind enjoy – and understand – stress.

 Breathing – the Building Block of Successful Stress Management

Most of the time we're unconscious about our breath. It takes place robotically. One of the handiest things you could do as you begin at the path to healing from Adrenal Fatigue Syndrome is to exercising deep, sluggish, easy and rhythmic breathing, using the diaphragm.

This permits release tension from the body, allows clear the thoughts, reduces fatigue and improves each intellectual and bodily nicely-being.

Balance Your Life

Too lots paintings, too much doing things for others, and too little time to take care of yourself. That's a recipe that has to trade for you to your recuperation to have a shot at achievement.

Get Rid of Energy Suckers

We've all said folks that appear to suck electricity out of the room whenever they're round. Got someone like that during your life? These human beings are strength-robbers, and you don't have enough power to transport 'spherical. Avoid them, in spite of the truth that best brief.

Happiness and Connections

And did you comprehend that happiness is a expertise, in location of an characteristic? Psychology professor and happiness researcher Sonja Lyubomirsky explains that simplest about 50 percent of a person's happiness is genetic. And of that fifty, high-quality 10 percentage is because of fitness, earnings and looks. Still, there's an entire 50 percentage that may be a located capacity.

Research tells us that one of the strongest indicators of happiness and genuine health is the exceptional and energy of our human connections. Relationships and circle of relatives, tremendous, but I'm speaking about network connections too. If you take a look at this and recognize that you've been spending all of your time being involved to your kids and cleansing the house, or giving the entirety you've were given to the workplace 12 hours a day, and you every so often spend any time without a doubt connecting with human beings on your network, now could be the time to start. What about your art work connections? They may be useful, but if the ones are the great connections you've have been given in your existence, it's sincerely worth taking every different look. Take a category. Join a club. Check out a network sincere or occasion. Find some thing that pastimes you, even a chunk, that your current time table doesn't appear to allow.

Go earlier and create time for a few romance, for some amusing with buddies and own family, and leave the guilt enjoy locked in the basement.

Look for techniques to spend quiet time with your self. Treat your self to a tub, a stroll, or a nail filing, a few component that you revel in, after which permit yourself to experience it!

 Lighten Up With Laughter

Laughter is one of the best sports for converting the manner we feel.

Studies display that those who snicker regularly have lower levels of cortisol and epinephrine, lower blood stress, and decrease feelings of tension and pressure.

The studies moreover suggest that even faking laughter is useful: the frame doesn't look like capable to differentiate most of the actual trouble and a synthetic snicker. No joking!

So, cross earlier. Let yourself chortle, notwithstanding the reality that it's miles at your self.

Exercise

It may be so difficult. On one hand, we recognize that we ought to get our heart fees up – cardio – as a way to stave off coronary coronary heart ailment. On the possibility hand, we understand that workout can precipitate an adrenal crash. We've been bombarded with messages about the importance of "on foot up a sweat", and we have been conditioned to suppose that if we haven't actually "driven ourselves to the limit", it wasn't in fact valuable workout.

With Adrenal Fatigue Syndrome, you want to alter all of that questioning. Exercise in reality has an important role in healing, however you want to create a method this is suitable to the quantity of Adrenal Fatigue Syndrome you're struggling with. Doing the wrong kind of exercising, at the wrong intensity diploma, can motive some other crash in area of assist you get higher.

The trick is to format a method and method that builds a customised software program that is appropriate in your particular degree of Adrenal Fatigue Syndrome.

Stop Intense Exercise

That's right. Stop any in depth shape of workout for as a minimum a month, longer if preferred. Take a ruin from cardio and all different varieties of strenuous exercise.

Restorative Exercise

Many humans with Adrenal Fatigue Syndrome will enjoy crashes brought about with the aid of regular stretching and strengthening exercise, that is often taken into consideration "slight" in the bodily health international.

Adrenal restorative exercise is unique, designed to assist find stability and restore health via connecting the mind and body in a nurturing and restorative way. If your Adrenal Fatigue is in the early stages, diploma one or , you may have fulfillment in restorative yoga training. For humans with greater superior Adrenal Fatigue, even restorative yoga can be an excessive amount of and reason a crash.

 Regular, Light Exercise

As you begin to heal, you'll likely discover you feel first-rate with strolling or mild cycling. Do not overstress your frame with strenuous sports activities.

You might also moreover additionally discover your self completely tired after workout, and as a surrender end result you've observed to keep away from it altogether. Completely understandable, but besides in some unspecified time in the future of an adrenal crash, it's now not a excellent concept to sincerely forgo any shape of exercise.

Chapter 7: The Road To Recovery

Adrenal Fatigue can soak up to ten years or more to appear, so it's far critical that you anticipate it to take the time to remedy, when you get on the right road to restoration.

Don't be discouraged if you don't shed pounds proper now. You want to do not forget that an Adrenal Fatigued body has endured a first-rate deal of stress and should heal first. Your organs and hormones need to be strolling optimally so as for weight reduction to arise. A gradual launch of weight will permit time on your frame to rebuild and consider itself all over again and, as a give up give up result, you may hold the burden off in the long run. Be affected individual and type to yourself, and allow weight loss to arise obviously.

You can also experience tempted to have an amazing time and lighten up when you begin feeling higher, but hold going! Your new way of life conduct are working. As time is going on, you can often lessen your dosage of nutritional nutritional dietary supplements and keep your newfound fitness through the strength of way of life and diet regime.

Recovery Process

Recovery pace and method is wonderful for nearly absolutely everyone with AFS. Depending at the severity of your unique state of affairs, distinctive fitness implications, and your willingness to trade, your method may additionally take a few weeks, some months, or maybe longer.

Preparation Phase

This training length is crucial for lengthy-term fulfillment.

•1 day to 6 weeks relying on the extent of AFS

•May be no sizeable improvement in signs and symptoms however the truth that nutrients are changing for the better

•Reactions to vitamins can also moreover upward thrust up, ensuing in feeling worse, modifications need to be made

•Body is in method of recovery and resetting internally.

Honeymoon Phase

•A few days to 12 weeks or extra relying on diploma of AFS

•Body handles strain better, decreased fatigue, anxiety particularly diminishes, sleep improves

•Can be mini-crashes and setbacks, don't despair, healing from those need to be quicker than earlier than you released into your healing avenue

•Energy starts offevolved to transport returned.

Plateau Phase

It's surely now not possible to set a time body for this era. It is probably some weeks or some months. It ought to closing for years and you may be truly symptom loose, if you have been in diploma one or of AFS.

But the reality remains that the body have to have time to rebuild itself, and for the ones in degree three or four, the greater advanced levels of AFS, this truely takes as a great deal time as it takes.

It is viable that the ones of you with greater excessive AFS may need to slowly adapt to a decrease diploma of normal strength function.

Expect Ongoing Cycles

Recovery isn't always linear. Like recovery from addiction, most important surgical remedy, or a few other most essential contamination, the direction of restoration is cyclical. Expect a spiral, and face up to the frustration or depression whilst you all of sudden feel which encompass you've suffered a setback.

I'll say it once more: cyclical mini crashes and recoveries are to be anticipated.

The most dramatic and terrific improvement can be in early levels of treatment. Then, after a term, you'll suddenly recognize that the setbacks have become an lousy lot a good deal less excessive, that they don't ultimate as long, and through the years, that the intervals among those mini-crashes gets longer. You'll word that your highs may be quite better, your lows now not as low.

Cycles, like a spiral, a bit improvement, a piece setback. Normal.

 Willingness to Change

All the incredible medical recommendation and assist in the worldwide will do surely no specific in case you don't examine the pointers. If you hold in conjunction with your horrible diet regime conduct, don't observe through on the exercising hints (both to exercising more, or a awesome deal tons much less, depending on your degree of AFS), and fail to take the advocated dietary dietary supplements, you could not see any improvement on your Adrenal Fatigue.

It furthermore takes a willingness to pinpoint and dispose of the sources of pressure to your lifestyles. This may be extremely hard, occasionally requiring the termination of long-reputation relationships, leaving a mission, or changing your relationship with money.

Not everyone exhibits they may be able to making the selection - choosing their fitness and well being over the popularity quo - but if you do, you'll acquire the rewards, experience higher, have greater energy and pleasure for your life. Speaking from private enjoy, it's miles well worth it.

Remember, you DESERVE to get properly, and also you DESERVE the time and energy to make it take place.

Feeling Like Yourself Again

If making a decision to walk down the street to recuperation, and you're taking to coronary coronary coronary heart the guidelines, recommendations and guidelines in this ebook, I recognize you can start to feel better.

You can also have your libido once more, your power once more, you could lose a few greater weight, and you may all once more have the strength and motivation to get through your day.

I even have travelled this street myself, and have in my opinion attempted the entirety I suggest here and greater. I even have researched and attempted a good buy more than is captured in this ebook, and I surely have located what seems to artwork, what doesn't, and what's without a doubt a waste of time.

I thanks for taking the time to have a look at this e-book, and I need you each fulfillment and real health.

Chapter 8: Presentation

The adrenal glands, positioned on top of the kidneys, are responsible for the secretion of important hormones: cortisone and adrenaline.

[You should not to be mistaken for cortisone, a metabolite from cortisol, with a comparative name, function, and genesis].

The adrenal glands and their hormone have number one physiological results on our body which encompass bone digestion device, metabolism, hormonal balance, gastro-intestinal function, thyroid capability, thoughts properly being, sugar stability, infection, immunity, and so on.

When the body research any big risk or catastrophe, our adrenal glands enhances the stress hormones, empowering us to comply to something task or catastrophe takes location to. At that aspect, whilst the emergency is over, the stress hormone subside and we settle without a doubt another time.

Today we live in a international that is suffered with this form of massive range of disturbing situations, that it is a help to apprehend that your adrenal glands serve various capabilities inner your body. Their crucial feature is that will help you reply and get via no matter all of the stresses.

We won't sense it usually, however strain is to be had in numerous methods which we aren't normally aware of: physical, emotional, highbrow, natural, immune, or any consolidation of those. Since your adrenal glands work in coordination collectively at the side of your body and thoughts, they may be capable of react to every form of pressure and anxiety.

An excessive amount of stress or anxiety can bring about overactive adrenal glands. This scenario is commonly stamped through dissentions of weakness, unsteadiness and memory loss. Other key manifestations include faded hair increase, chills or today's feelings of being bloodless, sustenance cravings and a failure to conform to pressure.

Overactive adrenal glands can be recuperated and restored to herbal potential via hold the food plan, herbs, regular adrenal-yoga (relaxation) sports activities and, most importantly, the selection of current strain and tension.

Overactive adrenal glands commonly create an additional of cortisone and in all likelihood different adrenal hormones. Since cortisone assumes a thing in growing sugar, this is ensuing inside the progressed blood sugar stage. About whether or not or not or now not, this will land up prompting situations like insulin resistance and metabolic disease.

Underactive adrenal glands, rather, stop result insufficient secretion of hormones, especially cortisone, to hold up harmony of organs in the body. A regular clinical problem with underactive adrenal organs is hypoglycemic signs and symptoms due to versions in the glucose diploma.

Ordinary, wholesome our bodies release cortisone to launch glucose to maintain up the talents of our involved system, organs and cells even as glucose ranges lower many of the food, or in a unmarried day for the duration of snoozing hours. At the issue at the same time as cortisone is distracted, glucose ranges get excessively low.

The adrenal glands discharge epinephrine as their natural affiliation. This causes the discombobulating, unsteadiness and crabbiness that human beings with low glucose experience, and is the purpose human beings with low glucose normally wake up in the various sleep inside the night time.

As our tension ranges lower the usefulness of our adrenal glands, so it influences particular capabilities in our frame.

Other than their important feature in managing pressure, your adrenal organs:

•Keep up the parity of in greater of fifty hormones in your frame

•Oversee stress and intercourse hormones and additionally diverse specific hormones which they find themselves able to harmonize

•Support in directing blood flow into strain and our coronary coronary heart fee

•Support in balancing glucose stages

•Calms aggravation at some point of the body organs

•Help sensory device capability (behavior, mind-set, memory, thinking technique)

As ought to be obvious, the adrenal glands are so cautiously interwoven with our physiological and emotional prosperity that we want to recollect what our our our bodies are letting us understand.

By know-how our our bodies and the detail that those small organs characteristic, there can be no motive in the again folks to enjoy the unwell results of weight growth, fluffy questioning device, a napping sickness, severe exhaustion, thyroid hassle, and speedy developing antique/maturing way.

The forms of stressors that decorate the adrenal organs include:

☐ Physical trauma

☐ Chemical pollution

☐ Poor food regimen

☐ Abundance/over Exercise

☐ Lack of sleep

☐　Infections

☐　Enthusiastic trauma anxiety (Depression)

☐　Wrong drugs

☐　Pregnancy

Biology of Adrenal Glands

Most people have had the enjoy in which they've got felt amazingly tired and depleted and afterward the bulk of a stunning each specific surge of electricity goes to their assist. In like way, while we experience dread and our coronary coronary coronary heart starts off evolved hustling the adrenal gland is freeing adrenaline and one among a type anxiety related hormones to address the primary characteristic and offer for us the greater assist of strength that we need to traverse the passionate pressure and tension.

When the mind deciphers an occasion as debilitating (distressing) the adrenals start to paintings. They flag the sensory machine to get geared up to fight or break out. This sign assembles the breathing and circulatory structures of the frame for crisis interest. Save power in the frame is known as upon, and capacities are redirected a protracted manner from elegant, homeostatic frame capability consisting of those of the immunity.

Despite the reality that the fight or get away reaction can be over, the immunity response permits the frame to hold preventing the stressor extended after the impacts of our sensory device have prolonged beyond off. When this usa of disaster is stored up for unrelieved limits of time, the body's stores gotten to be exhausted and the immunity is debilitated. Long and constant over-enactment of these hormones can damage the kidneys and adrenal glands, obstructing the functionality of the immune device to function.

When adrenal capability is disabled or feeble, an person can also moreover experience the ill outcomes of low blood sugar, low pulse charge, low body temperature, and an mixture feeling of depletion. At the issue whilst anxiety is drawn out the organs begin to debilitate and distinctive well-being related issues can set in, as an example, hypoglycemia.

A percent of the normal problems that beautify adrenal weariness are resulted with tension, pressure, lousy diet, over-utilization of sugar and eating sensitive carbs, abuse of perk, liquor, wrong medicinal pills, nicotine, and weight-reduction plan B and C insufficiencies.

As such the body responds the same approach to every real and anticipated dangers. For instance, unrelieved agonizing over losing your technique can bring about the same over-saddling of the adrenals and the resultant concealment of the immunity as sincerely dropping your technique.

If an individual succumbs successfully to anaphylaxes and ailments, feels usually emptied and depleted, research low glucose and immoderate blood stress, after which the frame may be frail adrenals.

A standout a number of the maximum conspicuous caution signs of adrenal glands deficiency is steady weak aspect. In a few sufferers, thyroid troubles cover adrenal problems. In those instances, the reputation of the adrenal glands and the thyroid glands want to be evaluated. The nicely timed treatment must be tried surely after this willpower is made.

Behavior of Sensitivities and intolerances for the right nourishments beautify the digestive system problems and discharging our sustenance accurately. This is the reason looseness of the bowels; constipation and one of a kind digestion issues are habitually the number one indications of a slender mindedness.

They likewise keep us from preferably digesting and soaking up all the supplements in our nourishments, abandoning us debilitated and coffee in strength. They can likewise decorate aggravation within the stomach, which triggers an arrival of histamine (along its warning symptoms and symptoms of sniffling and hacking). Ultimately, thru preserving us from digesting our nourishment legitimately they may likewise sell the improvement of unwanted microbes in our belly, debilitating our immune machine an awful lot greater.

There are some easy strategies to manipulate nourishment intolerances and sensitivities. Here are a number of the guidelines for reference.

•Avoid the nourishment being noted. If you have had been given a snug thought of which nourishments are bringing about you issues, be extra careful in warding off them! If you do no longer understand past any doubt, you can have a flow into at disposing of each one in flip, for a time of a week, till you've got diagnosed the wrong nourishment. Sustenance affectability trying out is furthermore a desire, but it does have a propensity to be very questionable. Depend on it for direction truly your reaction to all sustenance is a considerably more dependable take a look at.

•Take nutritional dietary supplements to reinforce your digestion. The most famous complement on this class is Glutamine, an amino acid that your intestinal inner surfaces use as a gasoline source. This allows inside the repair and restoration of the intestinal coating. You can likewise try demulcent herbs like licorice or elusive elm, which act to cover the intestinal protecting and ensure it from aggravations.

•Take herbal nutritional nutritional dietary supplements to enhance your digestion. If you aren't digesting sustenance nicely, and experiencing aspect effects like bloating, gasoline, loose bowels or constipation, taking digestive catalysts (digestive enzymes) can provide help. They will allow you to digest sustenance greater efficiently and take within the nutrients from the nourishment as well.

Chapter 9: The Adrenal Fatigue Recovery Diet

Keep away from more utilization of sugar. Refined carb, adrenal stimulants, and liquor have to be stayed faraway from. Fasting and cleaning ought now not to be utilized at the start of adrenal fortifying. The diet plan have to be a constructing and fortifying ingesting plan. Consume loads of clean and slowly steamed veggies and their juices as they consist of minerals to expect exhaustion.

In reclamation of the adrenal glands function, generally one must include potassium rich sustenance and stay away from nourishments which can be excessively excessive in sodium. This will help to hold the sodium/potassium stability inside the frame.

In the Standard American Diet (S.A.D.) eating plan, humans with the useful aid of and massive use up an additional of sodium, that would improve pulse price. If your frame is excessively excessive in potassium then lessening the sum you are devouring and add a bit sea salt on your weight-reduction plan. Don't upload salt on your ingesting plan in case your blood pressure strain is over a hundred twenty/80.

What you eat is in particular essential at the same time as you're enhancing from adrenal fatigue, a circumstance that exists at the same time as your frame's adrenal glands get to be depleted in view of lengthy haul, consistent stress and anxiety.

Nutritious nourishment is a key component to an powerful healing. Certain nourishments and add-ins want to be in your menu of dinners, consisting of these which might be excessive in wholesome protein and fats, nutrients, minerals, fiber and amino acids.

You can embody any of those menus of suppers as indicated by way of your inclination, however as a current guiding precept, consist of healthy protein, fats and starches with every supper.

Breakfast

Don't bypass breakfast if you have adrenal fatigue, and eat by using 10 a.M. As an method to maintain your glucose balanced. Abstain from eating culmination of immoderate sugar for breakfast in mild of its terrible impact for your blood sugar.

Your breakfast menu can include eggs, healthy fat (Oil, Nuts&Seeds) and greens. A advised clean menu lineup is eggs cooked in coconut oil alongside steamed broccoli or spinach. An change superb and filling menu preference is a smoothie containing eggs or protein, butter or ghee, coconut oil, and cinnamon.

Lunch

Make a time table to take the lunch with the useful resource of spherical twelve and near or 3 hours while you eat breakfast, even as you're recouping from adrenal fatigue. A menu opportunity is a huge green salad that includes verdant lettuces, cucumbers, celery, onions, garlic, radishes and tomatoes.

You can encompass hard boiled eggs, crude nuts, sunflower seeds and pumpkin seeds. Incorporate quinoa, lentils or rice with this lunch, with olive oil and new lemon squeeze as a dressing.

Dinner

Make a meal time via round 6 or 7 p.M. When you've got adrenal fatigue. Your menu ought to consist of correct first-class, supplement thick protein, as an instance, tempeh, tofu or beans salad with hemp seeds.

Avoid nourishments which might be fried or difficult overwhelming and hard to digest. Alongside healthy protein, include veggies, as an instance, inexperienced greens, broccoli or zucchini. Likewise include healthy fats, for instance, olive oil or flax oil on some of green salads.

Snacks

When you've got got got adrenal fatigue, do no longer preserve up lengthy in among suppers or snacks. This keeps your energy step up and your glucose tiers stable. You may sense pleasant while you devour something within to three hours.

A healthy, assisting nibble can be a handful scoop of uncooked nuts, gave which you are not oversensitive to nuts. An alternate brisk and supporting nibble choice is a hard-boiled egg alongside some raw vegetable quantities.

Suggestions:

Consume the more a part of your suppers in a smooth and comfortable surroundings, and make sure you chunk all nourishment properly and slowly. Doing these gadgets enables your frame to better digest and maintains the nutrients in sustenance. Avoid sustenance to which you are unfavorably prone, as ingesting these may be in particular difficult on your frame if you have adrenal fatigue.

If you're unsure what sustenance effects negative or hypersensitive responses, ask your properly-being medical doctor to perform a sustenance hypersensitive reaction check. Avoid sugars, perk, processed sustenance, junk nourishment and speedy meals out of your supper menus. Beverage sifted or spring water with easy lemon or its cuts collectively along with your suppers. You can likewise pleasure in herb teas, as an instance, warm or chilled peppermint or ginger tea.

Nutrients:

It is also extremely good to encompass calcium, Vitamin C, Vitamin A, and magnesium rich nourishments on your weight loss program. These nourishments assist calm the nerves inside the route of tension.

Calcium, Vitamin A, and Vitamin C rich sustenance encompass: Carrots, broccoli, kale, parsley, turnip veggies, collard veggies, Swiss chard, egg yolk, oranges, grapefruit, cantaloupe, cherries, pink and green peppers, and tomatoes.

Magnesium Rich nourishments encompass: Blackstrap molasses, sunflower seeds, entire grains, almonds, pecans, hazelnuts, and oats, tan rice, millet, white and pink beans, rice, beet vegetables, lentils, lima beans and peaches.

00004.Jpeg

Stay a ways from fast food consuming places and do not get processed sustenance. Avoid the donuts and precise baked gadgets at the identical time as minimizing coffee coffee consumption. Abundance of caffeine especially stresses the adrenals physiologically.

Make fantastic your vitamins D blood stages are above traditional. Anxiety and stress reasons the abundance of cortisol contrarily influences absorption of nutrition D.

There is plant sustenance that you may include to offer for you complete proteins if you're a veggie lover. If no longer, in any event keep away from processing packed meat gadgets. Make certain your nutrients intake is immoderate, specifically magnesium.

Begin Primal nourishment. Promptly begin a Primal or Paleo food plan. This exempts grains, vegetables, diffused sugar and vegetable oils, all sustenance that stresses the adrenals and builds inflammation.

Adrenal fatigue exhausts salt tiers inside the frame because it lessens aldosterone, the salt regulating hormone. Since enough sodium within the blood is needed for regular pulse charge, we are able to revel in discombobulating whilst aldosterone tiers drop.

Most people with adrenal exhaustion long for salt. Expend to the amount that salt as you could go through. Generously salt all of your nourishments and upload a squeeze of salt to any tea or water you drink. Utilize without a doubt Himalayan salt, Celtic sea salt, and now not processed salt.

Never, ever skip a supper with adrenal fatigue. This isn't always the time to exercising peculiar fasting! Your body isn't always able to accurately balance salt and glucose tiers in your blood, so you need to deliver those components frequently. Consume some thing little at normal periods. A small nibble should contain salt, saturated fats, and a healthful starch.

Chapter 10: Adrenal Nourishment With The Required Nutrients

The adrenal glands make use of more vitamins C than different organ or organ in the body. Vitamin C is critical to provide adrenal gland hormones. Thus, when you've been more forced, your adrenals may also have fed on vitamins C of the frame. A everyday dosage to help with adrenal stress is 1000 to 2000 mg.

Ayurved is the Indian manifestation of natural solution with a few thousand years antique information. Experts of Ayurvedic solution propose ashwagandha it's miles likewise mentioned. Ashwagandha is a tonic for exhaustion and depletion, reminiscence loss, muscle troubles, and unique facet consequences of adrenal weariness and fatigue. It can stability and normalize adrenal glands hormones.

To consume nourishments of the desired vitamins for Adrenal glands:

Almonds, Avocados, Yams, Swiss-chard, Parsley, Brazil Nuts, Kale, Walnuts, Oranges,

Lemons, Kidney Beans, Celery, Squash, Millet, Dried figs, Seafood (together with Kelp),

Berries, Hemp seeds, Dried dates, and Shiitake mushrooms (restoration mushrooms).

Herbs:

If our adrenals were suffered to long term strain, herbs can be useful in restoring and getting higher its healthy feature collectively with the proper food plan.

Licorice root has been applied for quite a long time to assist adrenal properly-being. It can assist cortisone ranges and manipulate the liver in processing them extra productively.

Sacred basil (tulsi) maintains up stability inside the frame's tension manner. It can likewise help adjust glucose and irritation degrees, that could have an impact on pressure degree.

Pau D'Arcy originates from a wild rainforest tree and is a maximum succesful tonic. It fortifies the immune device, in particular from tension and exhausted adrenals and might help the frame keep in addition harm from contagious, bacterial and viral ailments.

Feline's hook is also a South American herb that might get higher the immunity and combat aggravation inside the body that is one of the essential additives in stress and anxiety.

Wild oats are immoderate in potassium and magnesium which can be motive for tension and might calm the sensory device and also the adrenal glands.

Goji berries are rich in various required nutritional dietary dietary supplements, including nutrients C, which is easy for anxiety decrease and adrenal well being.

Schisandra berries have versatile houses, significance they do what your frame desires maximum. They upgrade the body's imperviousness to stretch uncommonly nicely.

Primal Recipes

Creamy Fruit Butter

A easy and home made creamy fruit butter recipe you may put together on your maximum cherished slight and sluggish cooker.

Ingredients:

four to five kilos pieces of fruit, cored and decrease

1/2 of to 1 mug unsweetened solidified squeezed apple pay hobby, separated

half of of teaspoon floor regular spice

1/4 teaspoon ground cloves

1/four teaspoon crisply floor nut-meg

half of of to 2 teaspoons floor cinnamon, separated

Squeeze of salt

Direction:

Place the quantities of fruit (for instance-apple) in a giant gradual cooker. Melt half of glass squeezed apple within the microwave or at the stovetop and spill over the quit end result. Sprinkle the end result with the all-spice, cloves, nut-meg, 1/2 of teaspoons cinnamon, and the salt.

Slowly aggregate with a great timber spoon. Place the top at the gradual cooker and cook on low temp for eight to 10 hours, or in a unmarried day.

Check the end result after eight hours. If they should be cooked longer, depart the sluggish cooker on. If the give up cease result are touchy, puree with an inundation blender while the pieces of fruit are nevertheless inside the sluggish cooker.

Alternately you may transfer them to a sustenance processor or blender and puree in little components. Taste and alter the flavoring, including the staying 1/2 of mug squeezed apple pay attention and 1/2 of of teaspoon cinnamon for sweetness, if sought. Keep on cooking on low with the quilt off until the creamy fruit unfold is thick.

Store in glass bumps within the refrigerator for 2 days, or forestall. To can, control in a water shower canner for 10 mins.

[Don't try peeling the pieces of fruit. The skin aides make a thicker creamy fruit butter and, once the fruits are pureed, you won't even know it's there].

Vegetable Curry with Chick-peas

Ingredients:

4 mugs cauliflower - reduce in florets

2 mugs Brussels grows - quartered

1 sweet potato - peeled and diced

1 pink pepper - diced

1 medium onion - diced

15 ounce cans chickpeas

15 ounce cans tomato sauce – of low sodium

½ cup diploma of mild coconut milk

½ mug chicken soup – of low sodium

1 tbsp cumin

1 tbsp curry powder

1 tbsp turmeric

1 tbsp cayenne

½ cup solidified inexperienced peas

Salt and pepper to taste

Plain yogurt, cilantro, sriracha and scallions

Chapter 11: Raw Nori Rolls

The rolls want a hint of arranging to set up the nuts and sun-dried tomatoes, but as quickly as the ones are organized, the relaxation of the dish meets up swiftly. These are excellent served proper away after they may be organized.

Ingredients:

1-half mugs crude almonds, soaked at room temperature water for eight-10 hours

1/3 sundried tomatoes, soaking wet four-6 hours

1 tbsp Smooth (or white)

2 tbsp crisply pressed lemon juice

1 tbsp tamari or soy sauce

1/4 tbsp black pepper

4 sheets nori (purchase untoasted if you want the ones to be altogether raw)

Vegetables for filling: carrot and cucumber sticks; floor deacon, meagerly lessen inexperienced onions, daintily reduce avocado

Salted ginger, as required

Wasabi glue, as required

Direction:

Set up the filling in a sustenance processor, hum collectively the emptied almonds and emptied tomatoes till you've got what resembles a first-class supper. Include the mish, lemon squeeze, tamari and pepper and system till the combination systems clean glue (encompass held tomato water if more fluid is wanted).

Set up the moves (you can utilize a sushi mat, however it a chunk lots), unfold spherical 1/four of the glue onto every nori sheet, leaving 2-three cm (1 inch) on the forestall.

Fill the cease near you with the segments of crisp veggies.

Saturate the vacant fringe of the nori sheet with water. Roll the nori into a protracted barrel over the veggies and around the empty component. Put on a plate or tray with the crease factor down; let it settle 5 earlier mins lowering into 8 uniform quantities.

Serve it with extra tamari, easy (cleaved) ginger and wasabi as fixings.

Vegetable Curry with Chick-peas

Fulfilling and consoling Indian propelled veggie lover dish full of protein and brimming with taste of warmth flavors.

Ingredients:

four cups cauliflower lessen in florets

2 cups Brussels grows, quartered

1 candy potato, peeled and diced

1 red pepper, diced

1 medium onion, diced

15 ounce cup chick-peas

15 ounce cup tomato sauce, of low sodium

1/2 of of cup moderate coconut milk

half of of cup fowl juices, low sodium

1 tbsp cumin

1 tbsp curry powder

1 tbsp turmeric

half tbsp cayenne

half of of cup solidified green peas

Salt and pepper to flavor

Plain yogurt, cilantro, sriracha and scallions trimmings

Direction:

Place veggies, chick-peas, tomato sauce, coconut milk, bird soup and flavors inside the slow cooker and hotness on Low temp for 8 hours or on High temp for four hours.

Before serving it, aggregate in green peas to heat.

Check for flavoring and conform correctly.

Serve over tan rice or grain of your choice with yogurt, cilantro and scallions. Sriracha is likewise an desire to encompass.

[Salt amount will rely on upon curry powder. You can use a without salt curry powder so you wound up including about ½ teaspoon of kitchen salt. In case you're not utilizing a without salt curry powder, you may require less].

Waldorf Inspired Kale Salad

Ingredients:

1/2 cup simple Greek yogurt

2 tbsp mayonnaise

1 tbsp crisp dill

2 little cloves garlic, minced

1 tbsp olive oil

3 tbsp fruit juice vinegar

1 tbsp agave nectar/honey

Salt and pepper to flavor

four cups broccoli slaw combination

4 cups cleaved kale (mixed and pressed)

1 cup shredded carrot

1 cup diced celery

half cup cleaved Gala stop result

Direction:

To make the salad dressing- blend Greek yogurt, mayonnaise, dill, garlic, olive oil, vinegar, and agave honey. Blend properly and season to flavor with salt and pepper and placed it aside.

In a huge dish, combine broccoli slaw, kale, carrot, celery and fruit. Place dressing over greens and mix it to mix. Mixed greens salad may be served right away or positioned apart inside the fridge. Greens salad is best consumed the equal day it is ready.

Relaxation Exercises

Oxygen consuming hobby consists of long term and moderate paced sports activities sports, for instance, taking walks, slight on foot, sluggish biking, and something particular manifestation of exercising that includes continuance.

This type of hobby will help reduce cortisol tiers and assist in burning muscle to fat quotients additionally. Oxygen consuming interest will gain the people who have suffered the adrenal glands issues within the early levels, wherein cortisol yield is excessive.

Adrenal YOGA

Yoga is a natural technological understand-a manner to enhance the proper features of the body, recognise the thoughts, and purify the soul. Experts will be predisposed to be extra adaptable, more potent, greater energetic, more slim, and additional younger, all of which can be attractive in Adrenal Fatigue restoration.

With exercise, you are fortifying and smoothing the sensory tool. It balances the useless tension response device persisted via the usage of most in Adrenal Fatigue. Blood float to inner organs is more potent, more oxygen is conveyed to the adrenal glands for mending; highbrow anxiety is cleared. Physical muscle agencies are advanced to make you greater glad, masses an awful lot much less on vicinity, and additional settled.

Since yoga's exercising benefits will increase on itself, it receives to be extra compelling approximately whether or not. It is proportionate to figuring out the manner to play a musical device, the extra drawn out you live devoted to it and practice the higher you get to be and the greater you got in pass once more.

Adrenal Yoga takes the exceptional of conventional yoga and alters it to healthful those with Adrenal Fatigue. For instance, tremendous extending and fortifying practices known as asana are uprooted, as they will invigorate the precise postures.

Benefits are exquisite with respiration strategies referred to as pranayam that may balance an arrival of adrenaline. Posture and lung capacity are better as is internal capability, lymphatic emptying, and the function of the immune machine.

Slowly one feels greater balanced and the body is higher prepared to go through tension of every day dwelling. Adrenal Yoga then, is ready restoring inner stability, and with parity, inner manage. It isn't approximately bodily adaptability, as numerous with Adrenal Fatigue are as of now very adaptable.

It is ready enhancing nice of the frame's natural functions, as some human beings are wholesome and though experience the ill effects of Adrenal Fatigue. Adrenal Yoga has the capability change liabilities, as an example, dread, powerlessness to relax, low vitality, anxiety, and depression, giving the person practicing extra manipulate and a greater balanced feeling.

Adrenal Yoga is precise of remedial yoga that is tenderly preserving with the aid of manner of the numerous postures. It places giant emphasis on frame mindfulness; musical adrenal respiration that is non stimulatory, valid postural association, and inclinations that tone muscles. Extra interest is about on slight and free actions which may be suitable for all, incorporating those which can be in advanced adrenal problems and conceivably close to being restricted to bed.

Science now may be familiar with that changing broken propensities is mostly a recall of the intellectual way. Adrenal Yoga facilitates through the usage of offering for you greater noteworthy manipulate of your thoughts and expertise of deceive it can play. This, maybe, is the issue that turns on a way of lifestyles trade. This is specially crucial in Adrenal Fatigue, while emotional stressors are the actual motive for the physical troubles.

Those with slicing place adrenal problems will mainly accept Adrenal Yoga and its transformational impact. Adrenal Yoga concentrates on upgrading and restoring parasympathetic stressful potential through way of showing the mind to struggle with the notion.

By easing off the variances of the mind, you can contact a extra extremely comfortable region inner. With exercising, you could get to be more privy to tranquility at your center at some level inside the direction of the day. It lets you apprehend that an entire lot of what you automatically get indignant and on element approximately isn't always that crucial.

It's nearly like toning down the dreary consciousness we have were given intuitively about beyond emotions of hatred, vintage glories, and stresses over what's to return once more. It locations our alarm, longing or abhor in a balanced issue of view that can be controlled in a methodical and coherent manner. It comforts us to live with the prevailing.

It brings down respiration and coronary coronary heart rate, complements (soothes) blood float to inner organs, as an example, the adrenals, digestive systems and reproductive organs, and permits you to rest and pay attention.

Some Adrenal Fatigue patients have simultaneous gastric and digestion problems. Adrenal Yoga enhancements the relaxation reaction and continues far from dynamic incitement of the perfect sports activities like backbends and pranayam method.

It brings down the quantity of cortisol while immoderate, and regulates the blood glucose levels. It does not squabble with technological facts but nutritional supplements technology. Adrenal Yoga consequently dietary supplements cutting-edge pharmaceutical's splendid with the beneficial aid of giving extra options to human beings in want of mending.

Adrenal Yoga is all encompassing attention on reinforcing your frame and mind. It bails you get the maximum out of some thing awesome forethought you get non-obligatory or ordinary remedy to your Adrenal Fatigue.

Chapter 12: Essential Yoga Postures

Sukhasana (Simple Cross Legs Pose) is bowing in advance, with brow and fingers resting on a cushioned seat. Stack clamped covers at the seat until you bought a comfortable posture. This posture releases pressure within the decrease lower back and neck muscle tissue, and feels particularly smoothing. If your legs aren't very tight, you can likewise embody similar ahead-bowing postures with one or each legs advanced right now whilst the forehead rests at the seat. Most humans need to raise the pelvis on one to three clamped covers even as rehearsing those postures.

Viparita Karani (legs up the divider, pelvis raised on reinforces or clamped covers). If the legs sense unwell of being at once, curve the knees and bypass the legs, with knees near the divider. This posture fortifies blood stress sensors in the neck and higher chest, activating reflexes that lessen nerve data into the adrenal organs, slight the coronary coronary coronary heart beat price, impede the mind waves, loosen up veins, and reduce the neither diploma of nor epinephrine circling inside the blood circulatory device.

While preserving your legs up the divider, improve your pelvis on enhance or clamped covers. As in step with yoga professionals, "If the legs feel wiped out on being at once, curve the knees and flow into the legs, with knees near the divider".

Breathing Process and Stress

Your breath can control your sensory machine. It lives as a great deal as expectations in every headings. Anxiety could have an effect to your breath. At the identical time your breath can likewise have an impact in your degree of tension.

At the factor while your sensory system is in a kingdom of anxiety, there are various changes that take place internal your frame. Your coronary heart rate will increase, organs amplify, veins agreement, and some extraordinary progressions take location.

Amid anxiety, your respiratory rate will boom, receives to be shallower, and also you inhale out of your pinnacle lungs, that is referred to as thoracic respiration or center fun. Fortunately, the association many of the sensory device and your breath likewise meets expectations in talk.

Your inhale is one of the scaffolds you have got available to govern your sensory machine. Your device for respiration tells your sensory device whether or not or not you're centered on or loose usa.

The respiratory strategies secured on this place had been confirmed to clean the sensory system. Correct breathing activities can be an important and loose part of your adrenal fatigue treatment plan.

Some Important Breathing sports activities to do at Home:

Abdominal Breathing

Sit without problems in a pass-legged role on the ground or flat lying in your returned in the corpse pose. Place the cushioning beneath the buttocks in case you need extra assist. Hands can be calm from the attributes otherwise you may vicinity one palm approximately the belly to truly experience that growing and falling. Relax the mind and frame.

Breathe in steadily and also deeply through the nostril, sensation your stomach growth and maintain the chest vicinity although. As you exhale, have a have a look at the stomach area sink down. Increase the stomach throughout the breath in and settlement the first-class stomach across the breath out. Exercise this particular exercising ten instances.

Breathing step by step and additionally deeply offers air in the direction of the lower a part of your bronchi and sports activities activities can also appreciably decorate breathing in and exhaling ability. It calms thoughts and frame, massages inner organs, calms inner mind and induces peaceful sleep.

Rib Cage Breathing

Sit clearly in a circulate-legged function on the ground or flat mendacity in your once more inside the corpse pose. Place the cushioning below the lowest in case you want a greater manual.

Place the palms on the edges with the bones at the way to feel all of them growing and also contracting. Lightly address the right belly, inhale slowly from the nose right away into your non-public rib cage.

Do now not pull the inhale sturdy without delay into your lungs; however maintain it centered among your ribs. Have the ribs growth outward and moreover the chest to be had even as you breathe in.

While you exhale, enjoy the bones agreement once more to the inner. Repeat it 5 instances. It calms the mind and the body in addition to tones up the lungs.

Alternate Nostril Breathing (Viloma & Anuloma)

Sit with out troubles within the bypass-legged characteristic on the ground. Keep the spine and moreover neck right away, however now not tight. Do no longer lean earlier. Place the useful useful resource under the buttocks or perhaps the legs in case you'd like loads greater guide. Place the left hand in your left knee.

Lengthen and stretch the thumb, finger in addition to pinkie (small finger) of your hand and retract decrease your certainly one of a type hands proper away into your very very own palm.

Start by the use of ultimate your non-public accurate nose together in conjunction with your thumb and also take a breath slowly thru the left nostril for a depend variety of eight.

After that press, the diamond ring and additionally pinkie palms in opposition to the closing issue from the nasal area, sealing the left nose near even as maintaining the thumb contrary to the proper nose, in addition to keep for a rely of eight.

Raise the thumb inside the proper aspect with the nasal location, starting the right nostril. Exhale slowly and moreover completely with the right nose for a recollect of eight.

Inhale slowly and step by step similarly to profoundly with the proper nostril, although preserving the perfect nonetheless left nose closed for the depend of 8. Cover the proper nose with the thumb in addition to preserve a depend huge form of 8.

Release the closing nose and additionally let out your breath thru the final nose for the rely number of 8. Repeat it five instances.

It calms and balances the mind and body, aids rest, will boom reputation, tones up respiration.

 To finish

For the right balance and particular health of Adrenal Glands:

Consume the sufficient amount of protein on your body!

You can verify the quantity to that you want utilising this protein programmer. Consume thirds of this within the morning and the closing zero.33 at lunch.

Go to mattress in planned time continuously and characteristic a snooze of 8 hours daily!

Your body is predicated upon on natural needs so waking and going to bed within the meantime every day will inexorably trade your electricity levels.

Consume daintily at night time time so your body can rest and revive on the same time as sleeping!

A incredible mixture for a quiet night time's sleep is mixture Pass greenery incarnate, Passion-flower and Chamomile. This ought to likewise help with that inclination of torpid in the morning. Drink a pitcher of water twenty mins previous going to bed.

Drink electrolytes to your water. A wedge of lemon want to do the assist!

Go easy on the stimulants. Attempt to stay some distance from touchy sugar or sugary juices as this worsens the susceptible factor over the long term.

Perhaps bits sensational but make a chamomile grass!

Lying in this kind of lawn and taking in its fragrance is wonderfully rest for the whole frame. On the opposite hand, placed four bunches of Chamomile or Jasmine vegetation/blossoms for your bathe, lie once more and lighten up.

Figure out a manner to like the forms of raw oats!

An change herb this is likewise an everyday sustenance is Avenal sativa, or oat. Taken as a herbal solution, it is a fashionable tonic for the nerves. Use uncooked oats wrapped in a cheese-material sack with the Chamomile/Jasmine on your shower for a notable skin soothing effects.

Chapter 13: What Is Adrenal Fatigue & What Causes Adrenal Fatigue?

Millions of humans around the area are suffering from adrenal fatigue, a scenario that many don't have any expertise of. The adrenal gland is extra or less the dimensions of a median grape. This little gland is chargeable for generating hormones which is probably important to the our our bodies wellknown characteristic. Things like blood stress, mineral stages and strain can be controlled thru those hormones. When the adrenals aren't on foot to complete capacity, it's miles referred to as Adrenal Fatigue or Adrenal apathy. Though this circumstance is getting increasingly interest, it's miles although now not identified with the useful resource of the clinical network as a real contamination. All the symptoms that go together with this illness can be defined via some thing else, because the clinical network says there may be no clinical evidence to lower back it as an true evaluation.

While now not as debilitating as maximum cancers or heart sickness, most people will revel in the bad signs and symptoms and signs and signs of adrenals that are not functioning properly, at the least once of their lives. Anything can reason the ones glands to surrender functioning properly. An contamination or a duration of top notch

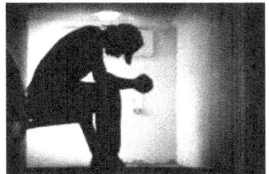

pressure or economic problems can forestall the manufacturing of the an entire lot needed hormone. There is not any sure age, race, gender or perhaps geographical place that has an inclination to be greater susceptible to this circumstance. Even if a person is noticeably healthy and receives an superb quantity of sleep and has specific eating conduct, they nevertheless could have troubles with their adrenals.

The adrenal glands sit on pinnacle of the kidneys. There is one on every kidney and a complete of in the body. The hormone that they produce is pretty crucial to our our bodies function. This hormone lets in alter the ranges of potassium, sodium and may even help hold someone calm during disturbing times. Yes, even the heartbeat is regulated with the aid of using the hormone from the adrenals. However, at the same time as this gland can do incredible matters for the body whilst it's miles functioning, it could come to be tired and gradual. When this takes vicinity the amount of hormones that it produces are inadequate and cannot hold up with the desires of the frame.

What Is Adrenal Fatigue?

Adrenal fatigue well-knownshows a chain of signs. When the adrenals are not operating well, the hormone isn't being launched inside the high-quality quantities. When the degrees of the hormone are off, then there are numerous signs and symptoms and symptoms and signs and symptoms that may arise. One of the most common reasons for the adrenals to save you operating is a period of extended and severe pressure. Nonetheless, it can additionally malfunction after a period of exceptional sickness or an contamination has wreaked havoc on the frame. Even a few detail as common due to the fact the flu can purpose the ones glands to be out of sync.

The problem is that many human beings have signs and signs and signs and symptoms that a few aspect isn't always proper in their frame, however they forget about about it; in location of having it checked out, they deal with it. The one aspect that is hard to triumph over with this case is the extreme feeling of exhaustion. A character who isn't getting sufficient adrenal hormones will enjoy exhausted maximum of the day, despite the fact that they have had a complete night's sleep. They can also additionally discover themselves taking naps or "hitting a wall" so to talk.

Is Adrenal Fatigue Real?

Adrenal fatigue is recognized most of the holistic or possibility medicinal drug practitioners. In massive, the medical network doesn't understand it as a health scenario. However, a tremendous deal is being accomplished to generate research and to alert medical doctors that this circumstance does exist. Remember Chronic Fatigue Syndrome? During the 1980's when this illness first came to slight, it changed into not diagnosed via way of the clinical network both. Today, there are tens of masses of thousands of people which can be identified each twelve months. In time it's far believed that the scientific community will spend some time analyzing and effectively identifying this circumstance.

Interestingly sufficient, the clinical community does understand that the adrenals can malfunction. For example, Addison's ailment is due to a problem inside the adrenal glands and in this instance, adrenal insufficiency is identified. The actual hassle is the shortage of medical proof that could deliver scientific doctors what they want. Holistic and opportunity medication practitioners use saliva tests, a few thing a conventional medical doctor usually doesn't. By combining hair sample, saliva, urine and blood tests, it's miles much less hard to get a more accurate picture of what goes on within the frame. Thankfully, there may be a brilliant deal of nutritional supplements which can be geared at those who gift with symptoms and symptoms of this overwhelming fatigue.

Signs of Adrenal Fatigue

Each man or woman may additionally additionally or may not enjoy the identical problems with this example. There are a few signs and symptoms that appear to always be gift, like exhaustion. However, holistic medical docs have located a bargain time and effort into the check of this situation. Some of the maximum not unusual signs and signs and symptoms notated are:

Exhaustion even after good enough sleep

Waking up tired

Needing to nap

Craving things which can be salty and candy

Needing stimulants, like caffeine, to keep going

Hair loss

Low blood strain

Can't overcome elegant ailments

Aches and pains of no precise nature

Having electricity in past due afternoons, none within the morning

Unexplained weight reduction

Difficulty strolling or keeping normality

Staying in mattress maximum of the time

Treatment for Adrenal Fatigue

Holistic docs have determined that the longer those glands are allowed to malfunction, the more harm it does. This circumstance may additionally come to be continual and can cause commonplace terrible fitness. When strain and steady infections are commonplace, they devise an appropriate surroundings to halt adrenal hormone manufacturing. By taking dietary dietary supplements which can be conducive to adrenal help and making some way of life changes, a affected individual stricken by this example can be handled. Eating healthful and getting the proper quantity of sleep and avoiding pressure are actually the begin.

Chapter 14: Who Is Susceptible To Adrenal Fatigue & How Common Is Adrenal Fatigue?

As noted within the preceding financial ruin, the signs and symptoms of adrenal fatigue have constantly been part of the regular human enjoy. It has best been in the past few a long time however, that the clinical community has understood the symptoms and signs and symptoms nicely enough to classify them into scientific lessons. Anyone with a nicely-walking adrenal tool is at risk of adrenal fatigue. This is especially right for healthful humans with a "move-getter" mind-set and a hectic manner of life.

The adrenal tool is accountable for intercepting alerts from the mind directing the discharge of hormones like adrenaline at some stage in periods of stress. Humans are capable of first rate feats of electricity, performance, awareness and cognizance. Prolonged periods of those types of stress can stretch the output of the frame's adrenal device beyond its genetically-decided "load limit." Though the spirit is inclined, the body might not be as lots as exceptional prolonged durations of physical

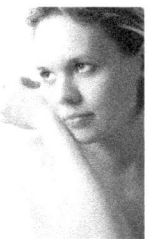

and emotional desires.

Whether it's far resulting from a deficiency of a selected diet or hormone, the body's adrenaline system can truly grow to be exhausted to issue in which a person might not gather the physiological gas to complete each day obligations. People experiencing adrenal fatigue may be aware a totally fantastic set of signs and symptoms and signs and signs that avert their normal feature.

Mental signs and symptoms of adrenal fatigue encompass the disability to popularity on obligations which is probably normally clean, a propensity within the route of outbursts of worry and unhappiness, and the dearth of hobby in preferred sports activities. Physical signs and signs include burdened sleep, shaking and tension, frequent bouts of contamination, and anemia. Adrenal fatigue is similar to an engine that is required to paintings more difficult and faster, however is disadvantaged of oil. No don't forget how tough it surely works, it's going to seize-up. Similarly, the human frame and thoughts will suffer damage and ache even as it's far overworked while being disadvantaged of the natural hormonal stimuli needed to effectively negotiate the demands of lifestyles.

Adrenal fatigue is particularly commonplace and might arise in any demographic. Adults, kids, and men and women of any race or social repute can enjoy the clinically-identified onset of "burn-out." In the beyond, adrenal fatigue changed into often burdened with melancholy and the archaic evaluation of Melancholy. Many humans honestly enjoy an over-taxed physiological country because of way of life options, inner chemical imbalances, or nutritional deficiencies.

The most ordinary symptom of adrenal fatigue is the thinking with the useful resource of an character of why they are unexpectedly feeling so poorly. People may ask themselves, "why cannot I get rested," or "why do not I ever experience happy at the identical time as my artwork is finished?" These people are correct of their perplexity. Humans are designed to perform a project and experience a amazing launch on the identical time as that task is achieved. This has been actual due to the fact that early man killed an animal for meals, tilled the soil, or ran circulate-u.S.A.

To supply a message. Modern people have to revel in that identical pride of entirety at the same time as searching after their households, finishing a mission at work, or growing a very ultimate fee on an exorbitant credit score score card bill.

When the pressure of living drains the frame's capability to provide sufficient wonderful temper hormones to interact with or experience satisfied completing sure duties; it's far a awesome indication that adrenal fatigue is the wrongdoer. Here are ten real existence examples of the feasible lifestyles of adrenal fatigue.

Every morning you wake a lot less rested and drink greater coffee. The caffeine stimulus does little to put together you for art work.

Normally, you sit up straight for outdoor paintings on the weekends. For numerous months, it's been a struggle to even placed your apparel on.

Instead of having prepared a favourite meal, your dinners have emerge as an exercise in using the microwave.

Your production at work is down with the aid of 30% clerically, or has emerge as risky if it is bodily exertions.

You come down with flu-like sicknesses or a cold as a minimum as soon as each extraordinary month.

You revel in unwanted weight advantage or loss, even though your weight loss program has no longer modified.

You begin to experience beaten in trivial topics concerning the troubles of own family individuals.

The pains to your joints and muscle groups do now not reflect your age.

Any desk bound sitting or popularity induces the out of control need to sleep, near your eyes, or mentally wander.

You have excessive shifts in slight sensitivity, mood swings at some stage within the night time hours and enjoy phantom pains to your limbs or extremities.

Adrenal fatigue is an indication that depletion of proper nutrients, relaxation and solace were absent in someone's lifestyles for lengthy sufficient to have an effect at the inner organs and glands that adjust how the body works. Many humans will envision the worst possible reasons why they will be feeling a whole lot less-than-proper sufficient. They will agree with a most cancers is growing, or they may be manic depressive, or their fortunes in life are geared towards failure and ache. In many adrenal fatigue instances, the ones emotions are a sign that an intensive intervention is wanted to "reset" the thoughts, glands and complete body to a degree wherein it can another time function typically.

In quick, adrenal fatigue is "burn-out" that is poignant enough to partially near-down the regular capabilities of a healthy body. The great manner to fight adrenal fatigue is thru session and prognosis from a scientific expert who acknowledges this illness's traditional symptoms. In tandem with different specialists like nutritionists, bodily therapists and cognitive behavioral specialists, physicians can help humans experiencing adrenal fatigue regain a right foothold on residing. It isn't uncommon that once adrenal fatigue has affected a person, that character will want expert assist and daily self-precipitated treatment plans to regain a modern day perspective. Thankfully, with deeper data of what adrenal fatigue simply is, anyone with this example can learn how to pinnacle off their personal "gas tanks" rapid.

Chapter 15: How Can I Tell If My Adrenals Are Malfunctioning?

Many are not wonderful of what is probably taking place to them once they begin to revel in really exhausted all the time, and sleep could no longer seem to assist. It makes completing every day responsibilities experience now not viable. Eventually, they will begin to marvel if their adrenals can be fatigued. It is just like many exceptional ailments, so it is able to be hard to inform for sure what might be wrong. This isn't a few element that is straightforward to discover, as it relates extra to how humans enjoy than a few issue resultseasily seen like a tumor. However, this situation may additionally additionally have a big effect on a person's everyday lifestyles.

There are many one-of-a-kind names that adrenal fatigue may fit via, which includes neurasthenia, hypoadrenia and adrenal apathy. Those who be by using way of it's going to find out that no matter how lots sleep they get, they may be even though really fatigued in the course of the day. They often describe feeling "grey" inside the direction of the day, and having to take pretty some terrific measures so that you can get the whole thing they want to completed. That have to encompass eating loads of strength liquids or depending intently coffee in fact to ensure that they've the power an excellent way to get via the day.

However, how do human beings realise if their adrenals are fatigued and now not some special trouble? Those who are wondering in the event that they might be stricken by this problem should recollect inside the event that they've skilled a number of specific signs. This can be feeling tired for cause, and in a way that isn't always fixed via getting a bit little bit of extra rest. Despite going to bed a first-rate time, the ones who have adrenal fatigue will discover that it feels almost now not viable simply to break out from mattress inside the morning.

Feeling in reality rundown isn't uncommon as nicely, and it is able to be difficult for humans to deal with. Many who be with the useful resource of this illness may discover that they may be crushed with handling this and all the extraordinary issues of their lives. People may additionally locate that they'll be getting ill extra frequently, and that they have a extra hard time getting properly later on. Also, folks that are dealing with strain in their lives also can find out that they may be in reality no longer able to deal with it the manner that they as soon as had been.